Cardiac Surgery Manual for Nurses
Orientation, Policy, and Procedures

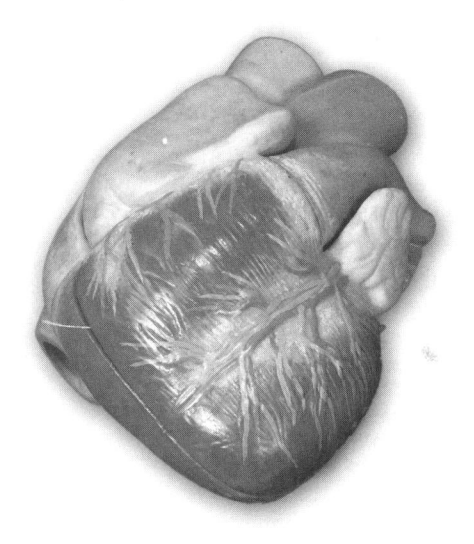

Debi Stephens-Lesser
Director
Cardiac Surgical Services
Fresno Heart Hospital
Fresno Community Regional Medical Center
Fresno, California

JONES AND BARTLETT PUBLISHERS
Sudbury, Massachusetts
BOSTON   TORONTO   LONDON   SINGAPORE

World Headquarters
Jones and Bartlett Publishers
40 Tall Pine Drive
Sudbury, MA 01776
978-443-5000
info@jbpub.com
www.jbpub.com

Jones and Bartlett Publishers Canada
6339 Ormindale Way
Mississauga, Ontario L5V 1J2
CANADA

Jones and Bartlett Publishers International
Barb House, Barb Mews
London W6 7PA
UK

Jones and Bartlett's books and products are available through most bookstores and online booksellers. To contact Jones and Bartlett Publishers directly, call 800-832-0034, fax 978-443-8000, or visit our website, www.jbpub.com.

> Substantial discounts on bulk quantities of Jones and Bartlett's publications are available to corporations, professional associations, and other qualified organizations. For details and specific discount information, contact the special sales department at Jones and Bartlett via the above contact information or send an email to specialsales@jbpub.com.

Copyright © 2007 by Jones and Bartlett Publishers, Inc.

All rights reserved. No part of the material protected by this copyright may be reproduced or utilized in any form, electronic or mechanical, including photocopying, recording, or by any information storage and retrieval system, without written permission from the copyright owner.

Production Credits
Acquisitions Editor: Kevin Sullivan
Associate Editor: Amy Sibley
Editorial Assistant: Patricia Donnelly
Production Assistant: Amanda Clerkin
Associate Marketing Manager: Laura Kavigian
Manufacturing Buyer: Therese Connell
Manufacturing and Inventory Coordinator: Amy Bacus
Composition: ATLIS Graphics
Cover Design: Kristin E. Ohlin
Cover Image: © Carsten Medom Madsen/ShutterStock, Inc.
Printing and Binding: Malloy, Inc.

Library of Congress Cataloging-in-Publication Data
Stephens-Lesser, Debi.
　　Cardiac surgery for nurses : orientation, policy, and procedures / Debi Stephens-Lesser.
　　　　p. ; cm.
　　Includes bibliographical references.
　　ISBN-13: 978-0-7637-4489-2 (alk. paper)
　　ISBN-10: 0-7637-4489-1 (alk. paper)
　　1. Heart—Surgery—Nursing.   2. Operating room nursing.
3. Surgical nursing.   I. Title.
　　[DNLM: 1. Cardiac Surgical Procedures—nursing.   2. Perioperative Nursing—methods.   3. Perioperative Nursing—standards.   WY 152.5 S824c 2007]
　　RD598.S74 2007
　　617.4'120231—dc22
　　　　　　　　　　　　　　　　　　　　　　　　　　　　　　　2006024164
6048

Printed in the United States of America
10 09 08 07 06   10 9 8 7 6 5 4 3 2 1

Contents

Preface	ix
Chapter 1: Introduction of the Cardiac Surgery Program and Team	1
Dynamics of a Cardiac Surgery Program	1
Cardiac Surgery Team	3
Standard of Care: Cardiac Surgery: Cardiac Surgical Team	9
Chapter 2: Staffing	15
Cardiac Surgery Policy: Staffing the Cardiac Surgical Suite	15
Cardiac Surgery Policy: Designated Cardiac Call	16
Cardiac Surgery Policy: Team Notification of the Elective and Emergent Cardiac and Cardiothoracic Surgical Procedures	17
Cardiac Surgery Nursing Procedure: Call Notification	18
Standard of Care: Cardiac Surgery: Staffing for Cardiac Surgical Procedures	19
Standard of Care: Cardiac Surgery: Cardiac Team Networking	21
Chapter 3: Education	25
Educational Program: Cardiac Surgery	25
Cardiac Surgery: Policy: Educational Requirements, Licensed Cardiac Nursing Staff	27
Cardiac Surgery: Policy: Educational Requirements, Nonlicensed Cardiac Nursing Staff	28
Standard of Care: Cardiac Surgery: Cardiac Surgery Orientation	29
Proficiency Skills Checklist: Circulating Nurse	32
Standard of Care: Cardiac Surgery: Proficiency Skills Checklist: Scrub Nurse	36
Cardiac Surgery: Policy: Monthly Cardiac Inservice Meetings	40
Cardiac Surgery: Nursing Procedure: Monthly Cardiac Inservice Meetings	41
Chapter 4: Scheduling	43
Cardiac Surgery: Nursing Procedure: Scheduling of the Elective Cardiac Surgical Procedure	44
Standard of Care: Cardiac Surgery: Scheduling of the Cardiac Surgical Prodecures	46
Cardiac Surgery: Nursing Procedure: Scheduling the Emergent Cardiac Surgical Procedure	48
Cardiac Surgery: Nursing Procedure: Same-Day Admission of the Cardiac Surgical Patient	50
Standard of Care: Cardiac Surgery: Same-Day Admissions of the Cardiac Surgical Patient	53
Cardiac Surgery: Policy: Scheduling Cardiac Surgical Support for Percutaneous Transluminal Coronary Angioplasty, Coronary Atherectomy, or Coronary Stenting Procedures	56
Cardiac Surgery Policy and Nursing Procedure: PTCA, Coronary Atherectomy, and Coronary Stenting Surgical Standby Support	57

Standard of Care: Cardiac Surgery: Percutaneous Transluminal Coronary Angioplasty, Coronary Atherectomy, or Coronary Stenting Surgical Stand-By Support   59
Standard of Care: Cardiac Surgery: Repeat Cardiac Surgical Procedures   62

Chapter 5: Case Management   65
Cardiac Surgery: Policy: Designated Cardiac Surgical Suite   65
Cardiac Surgical Suite   66
Cardiac Surgery: Policy: Organization of Supplies and Equipment in the Cardiac Surgical Suite   68
Cardiac Surgery: Nursing Procedure: Cardiac Surgical Suite Organization   69
Standard of Care: Cardiac Surgery: Cardiac Surgical Suite Organization   70
Standard of Care: Standard Cardiac Surgical Equipment   72
Cardiac Surgery: Policy: Preparation of the Sterile Field   74
Cardiac Surgery: Nursing Procedure: Preparation of the Sterile Field   75
Standard of Care: Cardiac Surgery: Sterile Field Preparation   77
Cardiac Surgery: Policy: Instrument Inventory Management   79
Cardiac Surgery: Nursing Procedure: Instrument Inventory Management   80
Standard of Care: Cardiac Surgery: Instrument Inventory Management   82
Cardiac Surgery: Policy: Cardiac Supply Inventory   84
Cardiac Surgery Nursing Procedure: Requisition of Cardiac Surgical Supplies   85
Standard of Care: Cardiac Surgery: Supply Management   87

Chapter 6: Preoperative Preparation   89
Cardiac Surgery: Policy: Perioperative Nursing Assessment of the Cardiac Surgical Patient   89
Physical Assessment of the Cardiac Surgical Patient   90
Cardiac Surgery: Nursing Procedure: Perioperative Nursing Assessment of the Cardiac Surgical Patient   95
Standard of Care: Cardiac Surgery: Perioperative Nursing Assessment of the Cardiac Surgical Patient   97
Cardiac Surgery: Policy: Preoperative Lab Procedures   100
Cardiac Surgery: Nursing Procedure: Assessment of the Perioperative Lab Procedures   101
Standard of Care: Cardiac Surgery: Preoperative Procedures   103

Chapter 7: Patient Care Activities   105
Cardiac Surgery: Policy: Transfer of the Stable Cardiac Surgical Patient to Surgery   105
Cardiac Surgery: Nursing Procedure: Transfer of the Stable Cardiac Surgical Patient to Surgery   106
Standard of Care: Cardiac Surgery: Transfer of the Stable Cardiac Patient to Surgery   108
Cardiac Surgery: Policy: Transfer of the Unstable Cardiac Surgical Patient to Surgery   109
Cardiac Surgery: Nursing Procedure: Transfer of the Unstable Cardiac Surgical Patient to Surgery   110

Standard of Care: Cardiac Surgery: Transfer of the Unstable Cardiac Patient
   to Surgery   113
Cardiac Surgery: Policy: Surgical Shave Prep for Cardiac Surgical Procedures   115
Cardiac Surgery: Nursing Procedure: Shave Prep for Valve Replacement/
   Repair Procedures   116
Cardiac Surgery: Nursing Procedure: Shave Prep for Cardiothoracic
   Surgical Procedures   118
Cardiac Surgery: Nursing Procedure: Shave Prep for CABG Surgical Procedure   120
Standard of Care: Cardiac Surgery: Cardiac Surgical Shave Preps   122
Cardiac Surgery: Policy: Continual Quality Improvement   123
Standard of Care: Cardiac Surgery: Total Quality Management   124

Chapter 8: Intraoperative Management   127

Cardiac Surgery: Policy: Physiologic Monitoring for Cardiac Surgical Procedures   127
Cardiac Surgery: Nursing Procedure: Physiologic Monitoring for Cardiac
   Surgical Procedures   129
Standard of Care: Cardiac Surgery: Physiologic Monitoring   131
Cardiac Surgery: Policy: Blood Utilization   133
Cardiac Surgery: Nursing Procedure: Bank Blood Acquisition   134
Standard of Care: Cardiac Surgery: Blood Utilization   136
Cardiac Surgery: Policy: Autotransfusion   138
Cardiac Surgery: Nursing Procedure: Autotransfusion   139
Cardiac Surgery: Policy: Stat Lab Protocol   142
Cardiac Surgery: Nursing Procedure: Maintenance of the Stat Lab   143
Standard of Care: Cardiac Surgery: Stat Lab   145
Cardiac Surgery: Policy: Surgical Skin prep for Cardiac Surgical Procedures   147
Cardiac Surgery: Nursing Procedure: Surgical Skin Prep for Valve Procedures   148
Cardiac Surgery: Nursing Procedure: Surgical Skin Prep for
   Cardiothoracic Procedures   150
Cardiac Surgery: Nursing Procedure: Surgical Skin Prep for CABG Procedures   152
Standard of Care: Cardiac Surgery: Cardiac Surgical Skin Preps   154
Cardiac Surgery: Policy: Positioning for Cardiothoracic Surgical Procedures   156
Cardiac Surgery: Nursing Procedure: Positioning for Cardiothoracic
   Surgical Procedures   157
Positioning for Valve Replacement/Repair Policy Unit: Cardiac Surgery:
   Nursing Procedure   160
Cardiac Surgery: Policy: Positioning for CABG Procedures   163
Cardiac Surgery: Nursing Procedure: Positioning for CABG Procedures   164
Standard of Care: Cardiac Surgery: Positioning for Cardiac Surgical Procedure   167
Cardiac Surgery: Policy: Draping for the Cardiac Surgical Procedure   169
Cardiac Surgery: Nursing Procedure: Draping for a Valve Replacement/
   Valve Repair Procedure   170
Cardiac Surgery: Nursing Procedure: Draping for the Coronary Artery
   Bypass Procedure   172
Cardiac Surgery: Nursing Procedure: Draping for a Cardiothoracic
   Surgical Procedure   175

Standard of Care: Cardiac Surgery: Draping for the Cardiac Surgical Procedure	177
Cardiac Surgery: Policy: Cardiopulmonary Bypass	180
Introduction to Cardiopulmonary Bypass and Myocardial Protection	181
Cardiac Surgery: Nursing Procedure: Institution of Cardiopulmonary Bypass	183
Standard of Care: Cardiac Surgery: Cardiopulmonary Bypass	190
Cardiac Surgery: Policy: Myocardial Protection	202
Cardiac Surgery: Nursing Procedure: Myocardial Protection Utilizing Cold Intermittent Cardioplegia	203
Cardiac Surgery: Nursing Procedure: Mycocardial Protection Using Warm Continuous Cardioplegia	208
Standard of Care: Cardiac Surgery: Myocardial Protection	211
Off-Pump Procedures	214
Aorta-Coronary Artery Bypass: CABG	216
Standard of Care: Cardiac Surgery: Aorta-Coronary Bypass Surgery	218
Cardiac Valve Surgery	226
Standard of Care: Cardiac Surgery: Valve Replacement/Valve Repair Surgery	228
Standard of Care: Cardiac Surgery: Cardiothoracic Procedures	236
Cardiac Surgery: Policy: Internal Defibrillation	243
Cardiac Surgery: Nursing Procedure: Preparation for the Use of Internal Defibrillation	244
Cardiac Surgery: Nursing Procedure: Intraoperative Defibrillation Technique for Patients Undergoing a Repeat Cardiac Surgical Procedure	246
Standard of Care: Cardiac Surgery: Defibrillation	248
Cardiac Surgery: Policy: Transfer of the Postoperative Cardiac Surgical Patient	250
Cardiac Surgery: Nursing Procedure: Transfer of the Postoperative Cardiac Surgical Patient	251
Standard of Care: Cardiac Surgery: Transfer of the Postoperative Cardiac Surgical Patient	255
Chapter 9: Special Procedures	**259**
Percutaneous Transluminal Coronary Angioplasty and Coronary Stenting	259
Standard of Care: Cardiac Surgery: PTCA, Coronary Stenting, and Atherectomy Surgical Support	261
Cardiac Surgery: Policy: Harvesting of the Internal Mammary Artery	264
The Internal Mammary Artery	265
Cardiac Surgery: Nursing Procedure: Harvesting of the Internal Mammary Artery	267
Standard of Care: Cardiac Surgery: Harvesting of the Internal Mammary Artery	271
Cardiac Surgery: Policy: Special Procedures: Slush Machine	274
Cardiac Surgery: Nursing Procedure: Slush Machine	275
Cardiac Surgery: Policy: Intraoperative Preparation of the Autotransfusion Pleural Drainage Unit	277
Cardiac Surgery: Nursing procedure: Preparation of the Autotransfusion Pleural Drainage Unit	278

Standard of Care: Cardiac Surgery: Intraoperative Preparation of the Autotransfusion Pleural Drainage Unit	283
Cardiac Surgery: Policy: Repeat Cardiac Surgical Procedures	287
Cardiac Surgery: Nursing Procedures: Repeat Cardiac Surgical Procedures	288
Cardiac Surgery: Standard of Care: Repeat Cardiac Surgical Procedures	290
Cardiac Surgery: Policy: Femoral Artery Cannulation	292
Cardiac Surgery: Nursing Procedure: Femoral Artery Cannulation	293
Standard of Care: Cardiac Surgery: Femoral Cannulation for Cardiopulmonary Bypass	295
Cardiac Surgery: Policy: Ventricular Assist Device Implantation	297
Cardiac Surgery: Nursing Procedure: Ventricular Assist Device Implantation	298
Cardiac Surgery: Standard of Care: Ventricular Assist Devices Implantation	300
Cardiac Surgery: Policy: Utilization of the Intra-Aortic Balloon Pump	302
Intra-Aortic Balloon Pump	303
Cardiac Surgery: Nursing Procedure: Intraoperative Placement of the Intra-Aortic Balloon	305
Standard of Care: Cardiac Surgery: Counterpulsation Using the Intra-Aortic Balloon Pump	309
Cardiac Surgery: Policy: Pacing of the Cardiac Surgical Patient	312
Cardiac Surgery: Nursing Procedure: Intraoperative Placement of Temporary Pacing Electrodes	313
Cardiac Surgery: Nursing Procedure: Insertion of a Permanent Pacemaker	316
Standard of Care: Cardiac Surgery: Pacemakers	318
Cardiac Surgery: Policy: Impantation of the Automatic Internal Cardioverter Defibrillator	320
Cardiac Surgery: Nursing Procedure: Implantation of the Automatic Internal Cardioverter Defibrillator	321
Cardiac Surgery: Standard of Care: Implantation of an Automatic Internal Cardioverter Defibrillator	323
Cardiac Surgery: Policy: Reimplementation of Cardiopulmonary Bypass	325
Cardiac Surgery: Nursing Procedure: Reimplementation of Cardiopulmonary Bypass	326
Standard of Care: Cardiac Surgery: Reimplementation of Cardiopulmonary Bypass	329
Cardiac Surgery: Policy: Re-Exploration of the Mediastinum for Hemorrhage	332
Cardiac Surgery: Nursing Procedure: Re-Exploration of the Mediastinum for Hemorrhage	333
Cardiac Surgery: Standard of Care: Re-Exploration of the Mediastinum for Hemorrhage	337
Cardiac Surgery: Policy: Intraoperative Mortality	340
Cardiac Surgery: Nursing Procedure: Coping with Intraoperative Mortality	341
Standard of Care: Cardiac Surgery: Intraopertive Mortality	344
Surgical Intervention of the Neonate	346

Chapter 10: Risk Management — 349
   Cardiac Surgery: Policy: Safety Reports — 349
   Cardiac Surgery: Nursing Procedure: Safety Reports — 350
   Cardiac Surgery: Policy: Housekeeping of the Cardiac Surgical Suite — 351
   Cardiac Surgery: Nursing Procedure: Environmental Control of the Cardiac Surgical Suite — 352
   Standard of Care: Environmental Control of the Cardiac Surgical Suite — 355
   Cardiac Surgery: Policy: Electrical Safety — 356
   Cardiac Surgery: Nursing Procedure: Electrical Hazard Prevention — 357
   Cardiac Surgery: Standard of Care: Electrical Safety — 359
   Cardiac Surgery: Policy: Electrocautery Utilization — 361
   Cardiac Surgery: Nursing Procedure: Electrocautery Safety — 362
   Cardiac Surgery: Policy: Protective Attire — 366
   Cardiac Surgery: Nursing Procedure: Protective Attire — 367
   Standard of Care: Cardiac Surgery: Risk Management — 369
   Cardiac Surgery: Policy: Surgical Consents — 371
   Standard of Care: Cardiac Surgery: Surgical Consents — 374
   Cardiac Surgery: Policy: Perioperative Documentation of Cardiac Surgical Procedures — 376
   Cardiac Surgery: Nursing Procedure: Perioperative Documentation of Cardiac Surgical Procedures — 377
   Standard of Care: Cardiac Surgery: Perioperative Documentation of Cardiac Surgical Procedures — 379
   Cardiac Surgery: Policy: Patient Transfer Report — 380
   Cardiac Surgery: Nursing Procedure: Patient Transfer Report — 381
   Standard of Care: Cardiac Surgery: Continuity of Care for the Immediate Postoperative Surgical Patients — 383

References — 387

Index — 389

Preface

Standards of care are devised for cardiac surgical procedures to provide guidelines of accepted practice for the caregiver, as well as clinical indicators in which to analyze patient care delivery and evaluate the patient's response to therapy. Standards of care include goals, expected outcomes, and nursing interventions relating to the assessment of the physiological, psychosocial, safety, and educational aspects of care.

The framework for these standards revolve around scheduling, staffing, risk management, education, case management, and special cardiac surgical procedures. These standards must integrate the cardiac surgical program structure; including the types of cardiac surgical procedures, customer identification, volume of cases, surgeon/anesthesia practice, and changes in technology.

The foundation on which these standards are built provides the stability to withstand variables that can change rapidly in this environment; including patient volume and case mix, resource utilization involving staffing levels and patterns, staff requirements for different cardiac surgical procedures, surgeon and anesthesia practices, anesthesia availability, emergent cases, procedure duration, patient acuity, and invasive cardiology procedures requiring surgical backup support.

These standards are also used to develop measurable criteria used to educate and assess the individual performance of the team member.

The following pages provide an introduction to these clinical standards. The beat goes on . . . by allowing the conduction of these standards of care, enabling a synchronized, effective pace conducive to a greater cardiac output!

Introduction of the Cardiac Surgery Program and Team

chapter 1

■ Dynamics of a Cardiac Surgery Program

I. Scheduling Modalities
   A. Cardiac/cardiothoracic surgical procedures
      1. Elective
      2. Emergent
   B. PTCA/Atherectomy/coronary stenting surgical standby support procedures
   C. Cardiac team notification process
II. Staffing
   A. Program analysis of staffing needs
   B. Job descriptions
   C. Daily staffing plan
   D. Call coverage
III. Case Management
   A. Time management analysis
   B. Cardiac surgical suite organization
   C. Instrumentation, inventory, and management
   D. Cardiac supplies management
   E. Special procedure protocols
   F. Patient transfer process
IV. Risk Management
   A. Continuous quality improvement program
   B. Safety
   C. Environmental control
   D. Universal precautions

   E. Regulatory compliance
   F. Intraoperative surgical documentation
V. Training Activities
   A. Structured orientation program
   B. Comprehensive training for the circulating and scrub nurse roles
   C. Cardiac surgery orientation manual
   D. Cardiac surgery clinical pathways
   E. Cardiac surgery/cardiac cath lab conduction pathways
   F. Perioperative policies, procedures, and standards of care
VI. Educational Activities
   A. Educational requirements
   B. Cross training
   C. Orientation process
   D. Monthly team meetings
   E. Monthly inservice meetings
   F. Competency review
   G. Cardiac surgery standards of care
   H. Policies and procedures
VII. Networking
   A. Service line approach
     1. Teamwork
     2. Expanded roles
     3. Standardization
     4. System review

Cardiac Surgery Team

The cardiac surgical team is an integrated group of professionals consisting of a board-certified anesthesiologist, a certified clinical perfusionist, two cardiac surgeons, two circulating nurses, and one scrub nurse or scrub technician. The staffing is structured to meet the daily caseload and provide 24-hour-a-day coverage for 7 days a week. These schedules are reviewed and adjusted, as necessary, to meet individual patient needs and unusual occurrences.

Cardiac Surgeons

There are usually two cardiac surgeons per cardiac surgical procedure. The cardiac surgeon(s) has been certified by the American Board of Surgery with additional training and or certification in cardiovascular/cardiothoracic procedures. The surgeon assumes full responsibility for all medical acts of judgment and the surgical care of the patient, including but not limited to the following:

A. Preoperative diagnosis and care
B. Selection and performance of the surgical procedure
   1. Communicates the patient's special needs to the team
   2. Supervises all personnel assisting during the surgical procedure
C. Postoperative management of care

Cardiac Anesthesiologist

The cardiac anesthesiologist works closely with the surgeon and perfusionist perioperatively with the continual assessment of the cardiac surgical patient.

Preoperatively, this professional evaluates the patient's laboratory values, pulmonary function, and overall physical status.

After the patient enters the surgical suite, the anesthesiologist establishes a peripheral IV along with invasive hemodynamic monitoring lines, that is, arterial and Swan-Ganz catheters. Continuous monitoring of pressures allows current assessment of the patient's hemodynamic status and needs, interpretation and location of pathology, provides early warning signs of possible cardiopulmonary complications, and enables the team to assess the patient's response to therapy.

Intraoperatively, before cardiopulmonary bypass, the anesthesiologist is responsible for the maintenance of the patient's airway and hemodynamic status, coordinating care with the surgeon and perfusionist.

During cardiopulmonary bypass, the anesthesiologist works closely with the perfusionist providing guidance for fluid replacement, anesthesia, assessment of lab values with the corresponding treatment, and administration of drugs.

After cardiopulmonary bypass is discontinued, the anesthesiologist retains control of the patient's ventilation and assists with the stabilization of the patient's hemodynamic status with fluids, drug therapy, or temporary pacing, if required.

Initially postoperatively, the patient is left intubated. The cardiac anesthesiologist accompanies the circulating nurse to the intensive care unit and leaves orders for assisted ventilatory control.

Perfusionist

The perfusionist is a board-certified professional responsible for the operation and maintenance of the heart–lung machine, stat lab equipment, and extracorporeal circulation during a cardiac surgical procedure. The perfusionist practices under the immediate supervision and direction of the cardiac surgeon along with coordination and communication with the cardiac surgical nursing team and anesthesiologist to facilitate the intraoperative management of the cardiac surgical patient. This professional is extremely knowledgeable of cardiac anatomy, physiology, and current technology related to cardiac surgical procedures. The perfusionist is responsible for evaluation of perfusion devices and equipment relating to safety, efficacy, and cost-effectiveness in order to meet the needs of the patient, surgeon, and change in technology.

Preoperatively, the perfusionist's job responsibilities include but are not limited to

A. Preparation of the perfusion circuits on the heart–lung machine that are responsible for the blood and oxygen exchange between the patient and heart–lung machine
B. Evaluation of the patient's cardiovascular history and lab values
C. Assessment of the patient's weight and calculation of the cardiac index and total body surface area needed to establish guidelines for the speed of delivery of blood through the extracorporeal circuits to provide adequate cerebral and peripheral perfusion
D. Baseline ACT determinations and dosage for heparinization
E. Distribution of the extracorporeal table circuits to the scrub nurse

Initiation of cardiopulmonary bypass is facilitated through the perfusionist. During cardiopulmonary bypass, the perfusionist monitors the circulation and ventilation of the patient, maintaining continual communication among the primary surgeon, anesthesiologist, and nursing team. The hemodynamic status of the patient is assessed and therapy instituted as needed to maintain an adequate cardiac output and tissue perfusion during cardiopulmonary bypass. The ACT levels are checked continuously, and heparin is given at intervals to maintain the blood at a safe level, preventing coagulation from developing in the extracorporeal circuits and vasculature structures of the patient.

The perfusionist is responsible for the type and amount of fluid volume replacement, dependent on estimated blood loss, HCT, ABGS, and arterial pressure measurements necessary for the regulation of arterial oxygen content, carbon dioxide exchange and renal perfusion. During cardiopulmonary bypass, he or she is also responsible for electrolyte balance and glucose control needed for cell metabolism, regulation of the patient's body temperature, and myocardial protection. The perfusionist also operates the cell saver and intra-aortic balloon pump as needed.

Weaning from cardiopulmonary bypass is a coordinated effort by the cardiac surgeon, anesthesiologist, and perfusionist. As the patient's hemodynamic status is stabilized and hemostasis is obtained, the patient is slowly weaned from the heart–lung machine.

Postoperatively, the perfusionist performs ACT and HPT tests to determine the protamine dose needed to reverse the anticoagulation effect of heparin. After the patient is hemodynamically stable, the circuits on the heart–lung machine are broken down and appropriately discarded. Any blood remaining in the oxygenator is hemoconcentrated through a special filter and returned to the patient, providing fluid replacement with a high hematocrit.

The heart–lung machine and stat lab equipment are cleaned and disinfected after each procedure. Perfusion supplies are organized for the next case.

The perfusionist fulfills all medical and legal requirements for case documentation during cardiopulmonary bypass and quality assurance checks on the stat lab equipment.

Assistance with transportation to the unit is provided, if needed.

Cardiac Circulating Nurses

Each cardiac surgical procedure requires a minimum of two circulating nurses. These nurses have defined roles that when working collaboratively facilitate case flow, expedite surgery, and promote patient safety. These roles are divided into a first and second circulating position.

The Primary Circulating Nurse's Role

A. General room assessment for the necessary equipment and functional capability
B. Preparation of the IV lines and invasive monitoring equipment
C. Retrieval of the appropriate narcotics and drugs for the anesthesiologist
D. Patient identification and assessment
E. Chart assessment for the pertinent consents and lab tests along with their values
F. Transfer of the patient from the gurney/bed to the operating room table
G. Placement of the noninvasive monitoring equipment: blood pressure cuff, EKG electrodes, and pulse oximeter

H. Assistance to the anesthesiologist during placement of invasive monitoring lines
I. Acquisition of blood from the blood bank, verifying the correct identification of the patient and blood with the second circulating nurse
J. Assistance with induction, PRN
K. Placement of the electrosurgical dispersement pads
L. Positioning the patient appropriately for the type of procedure to be performed, usually with arms tucked at the patient's sides, with the assistance of the second circulator. If a radial artery harvesting is to be done, the operative arm is positioned and secured on an armboard.
M. Positioning the birdcage over the head of the bed with the assistance of the second circulator
N. Completion of the surgical prep with the assistance of the second circulator
O. Connection of equipment from the sterile field
P. Communication of intraoperative information to significant others and members of the healthcare team
Q. Psychological and physiological monitoring of the individual with continual evaluation of outcomes in relationship to nursing activities
R. Case documentation
S. Performs the required sponge, instrument, and needle count with the scrub nurse
T. Converts the cell saver reservoir to the autotransfusion/pleural drainage system or connects chest tube drainage unit to suction
U. Transfers the postoperative patient to the intensive care unit with a thorough report of the procedure performed and the immediate status of the patient
V. Returns blood to the blood bank
W. Helps clean and restock the cardiac surgical suite

The Second Circulating Nurse

The second circulator is an assistant to the first circulator and the first scrub nurse. After the surgical prep is completed and the equipment from the sterile field is connected, the second circulator also functions as a second scrub nurse.

This role includes the following but is not limited to the following:

A. Assists the first circulator in the overall room preparation
B. Assists the first scrub nurse/tech with the preparation of the sterile field by opening the sterile supplies and instruments
C. Counts needles, instruments, and sponges with the first scrub nurse/tech
D. Pours saline for the slush machine and gives the scrub nurse/tech the necessary solutions and medications needed on the sterile field
E. Inserts the bladder catheter while the first circulator is positioning the arms and placing electrosurgical dispersement pads

F. Assists the first circulator with the surgical prep and equipment connections from the sterile field
G. If the surgical procedure is a CABG, functions as a second scrub nurse and assists with the conduit harvesting. If it is a valve procedure requiring a porcine valve, the second scrub nurse/tech washes the valve.
H. After the vein harvesting is completed, the second scrub nurse/tech changes gloves, covers the legs with a drape, and assists the first scrub nurse/tech to move into position over the patient's legs. The second scrub nurse/tech then holds the heart as needed to provide exposure during the revascularization of the coronary arteries.
I. When the second scrub role is completed, the nurse/tech breaks scrub and assists the first circulator for the duration of the case.
J. Give breaks or lunch relief, as needed
K. Assists the first scrub nurse/tech with the instrument and equipment decontamination at the end of the case
L. Restocks the cardiac surgical suite

The Primary Scrub Nurse/Tech

The primary scrub nurse or tech has an integrated knowledge of cardiac anatomy and physiology, cardiac surgical procedures, hemodynamic parameters, mechanics and function of the heart–lung machine, the physics of cardiopulmonary bypass, along with physician practices and changes in technology relating to cardiac surgery. This scrub nurse/tech prioritizes actions in response to the changing hemodynamic status of the patient to meet the surgeon's needs. This nurse/tech is a resource person for the special needs of the surgeon.

This defined role includes the following:

A. Acquisition of the pertinent supplies, equipment, instrumentation, and suture needed at the sterile field
B. Preparation of the sterile field
C. Sponge, needle, and instrument counts, preop, and closing
D. Gowning/gloving of the surgeons
E. Assists with the draping procedure
F. Assures that all equipment coming from the sterile field is operational
G. Inspects instruments for proper functioning
H. Organizes the extracorporeal table circuits and passes the appropriate ends off to the perfusionist at the appropriate time to connect to the heart–lung machine extracorporeal circuits
I. Assists the surgeon with the cannulation process for cardiopulmonary bypass and ensures that the heparin is given before initiation of cardiopulmonary bypass

J. Assists in the revascularization or valve replacement/repair procedures by passing the necessary instruments and sutures
K. Handles and cares for the vein grafts/valve before implantation
L. Communicates the needs of the patient or surgeons to the circulating nurses
M. Assists with the room cleanup and returns instruments to central supply for the decontamination process
N. Keeps the physician's preference cards updated
O. Restocks the cardiac surgical suite
P. Ensures that another cardiac surgical case of supplies and instruments are organized on a cart and in the cardiac surgical suite, ready for another case

Coordinated teamwork with clear, concise communication is essential for the delivery of quality care in the cardiac surgery environment. Each job role has individual responsibilities that overlap, promoting versatility and flexibility during emergent situations, enabling continuity of care when seconds count.

Standard of Care: Cardiac Surgery: Cardiac Surgical Team

I. Cardiac Team Members
   A. Cardiac surgeons
      1. Primary—must be certified or eligible for certification by the American Board of Thoracic Surgery or the American Board of Surgery with training and experience in cardiovascular procedures
      2. Assistant
      3. Physician assistant, if applicable
   B. Cardiac anesthesiologist—must be certified or eligible for certification by the American Board of Anesthesiology
      1. Anesthesia—airway maintenance
      2. Invasive line placement
      3. Maintenance of hemodynamic parameters
      4. Coordination of patient care with perfusionist and surgeon
      5. Transport of the patient to the intensive care unit
      6. Anesthesia case documentation
   C. Perfusionist—must be certified or eligible for certification and practice under the immediate supervision of a cardiac surgeon
      1. Operation of the heart-lung machine and related perfusion equipment
      2. Stat lab
      3. Perfusion supplies
      4. Operation of the intra-aortic balloon pump
      5. Coordination with the cardiac manager to facilitate the intraoperative care of the cardiac surgical patient
   D. Hemodynamic monitoring specialist
      1. IV fluids and drug preparation
      2. Transducer/transducers preparation, calibrating, and troubleshooting
      3. Assistant to the anesthesiologist
      4. Autotransfusion operation
      5. Operation of the intra-aortic balloon pump
      6. Transport of the patient to the intensive care unit with transfer of invasive lines
   E. Nursing staff
      1. Two registered nurses, one surgical technician, or three registered nurses
         a. Primary circulator

1. Assists the first scrub nurse in the preoperative room preparation
2. Locates the hospitalized patient and sends for him or her at the appropriate time
3. General room preparation, with assessment of and acquisition of the appropriate equipment necessary for the cardiac surgical procedure
4. Identification of the patient, completion of the preoperative surgical checklist, transfer of the patient to the surgical table, and positioning for the surgical procedure
5. Perioperative plan of care for the individual cardiac surgical patient
6. Placement of noninvasive monitoring equipment; blood pressure cuff, cardiac electrodes, pulse oximeter probe
7. Placement of the electrosurgical dispersement pad(s)
8. Completion of the surgical skin prep
9. Coordinates the intraoperative needs for the patient, surgeon, anesthesiologist, perfusionist, and scrub nurse
10. Documentation of the surgical event
11. Coordinates pertinent communication to the intensive care unit and family
12. Assists with the transport of the patient to the intensive care unit
13. Assists with the surgery suite housekeeping and the restocking of room supplies

b. Second circulator
1. Coordinates the intraoperative care with the primary circulator
2. Completes the required sponge, needle, and instrument counts with the scrub nurse
3. Coordinates the transfer of the blood from the blood bank to the operating room, verifying correct patient identification with the amount of blood available
4. Assists the scrub nurse in case preparation, as needed
5. Functions in a second scrub role, as needed
6. Assists the circulator for the duration of the case
7. Assists with relief of the circulator or scrub nurse, as needed
8. Assists with the safe transport of the patient from the surgery table to the bed
9. Returns the unused bank blood to the blood bank

   10. Assists with the surgical suite housekeeping after the case is completed and helps with restocking of room supplies
  c. Primary scrub nurse
   1. Assists the circulating nurse in the preliminary housekeeping duties
   2. Responsible for organizing the appropriate instrumentation and supplies according to the physician's preference and procedure to be performed
   3. Accountable for the preparation and maintenance of the sterile field
   4. Prepares suture and performs the required sponge, needle, and instrument counts at the appropriate intervals
   5. Prioritizes actions to meet the needs of the patient and surgeon
   6. Works collaboratively with the perfusionist in securing and maintaining the extracorporeal circulation circuits from the sterile field to the heart–lung machine
   7. Communicates the surgeon/patient's needs to the circulator, as needed
   8. Assists in the transfer of the patient from the surgical table to the unit bed after completion of the surgical procedure
   9. Separates the dirty instruments, according to hospital policy, and sends them to the instrument reprocessing area after the patient has left the surgical suite
   10. Organizes the supplies and instrumentation needed for the next case

F. Cardiac manager
 1. Responsible for team development
  a. Liaison between the cardiac surgeons and the team members
  b. Liaison between the anesthesiologists and team members
  c. Liaison with administration
  d. Staff selection and mix
  e. Training of staff members; skills checklist
  f. Monthly staff meetings
  g. Staff scheduling, both regular working hours and call coverage
  h. Staff job performance evaluations
  i. Liaison with the units related to cardiac services
 2. Cardiac surgery budget management
  a. Assessment for the budget
   1. Historical data
   2. Changes in patient population

3. Changes in services
4. Changes in composition of the medical staff
5. Changes in delivery of healthcare service
6. Changes in nursing practice
7. Impact of regulatory agencies
8. Fiscal impact of trends
   b. Completion of a budget every fiscal year
      1. A developed action plan setting priorities and schedules for the procurement of human resources, equipment, and supplies
      2. Monthly productivity and budget compliance review and evaluation
      3. Evaluation of pay practices with flexible staffing to meet case demands
      4. Cost/charge models for valve replacement/repair and coronary artery bypass procedures
   c. Management of cardiac surgical supplies and inventory
      1. Custom packs
      2. Suture
      3. Valve inventory
      4. Intra-aortic balloons
      5. Special cardiac supplies
      6. Instrumentation
      7. Instrument and supply locator file for quick reference
3. Heart team notification
   a. Scheduled cardiac procedures
   b. Emergent cardiac procedures
   c. PTCA, coronary arthrectomy and stenting coverage
4. Continual quality management
   a. Perioperative case documentation
      1. Operative record
      2. Fluid utilization sheet
      3. Procedure log
   b. Pertinent data collection
      1. Valve/implant log
      2. Special orders' log
      3. Documentation of type of electrical equipment, with a log of maintenance and inspection
      4. Housekeeping documentation log
      5. Monthly cardiac staff meetings, agendas, and attendance records

        6. Monthly safety reports
- c. Review and revision of cardiac surgical procedures and policies as needed
    1. Updating the physicians' preference cards
    2. Establishing standards of care with quality indicators for evaluation of care rendered
    3. Documentation of variances with follow-up evaluation

Staffing

chapter 2

■ Cardiac Surgery Policy: Staffing the Cardiac Surgical Suite

Cardiac surgery's policy is to provide staff for the cardiac surgical suite 24 hours a day, 7 days a week. After hours—nights and weekends—are covered by "on-call" hours, with a call team assigned by the cardiac manager. The staffing is organized to incorporate a multidisciplinary team to facilitate open-heart surgery. The staffing schedules are reviewed and adjusted as necessary to meet defined patient needs and unusual occurrences.

Staffing for each cardiac case shall consist of but not be limited to the following:

1. Two circulating nurses
2. One scrub nurse
3. Perfusionist
4. Hemodynamic monitoring technician/anesthesia assistant
5. Cardiac anesthesiologist
6. Cardiac surgeons
7. Physician's assistant (optional)

Cardiac Surgery Policy: Designated Cardiac Call

Cardiac surgery's policy is that after-hours staffing for cardiac surgery be covered with an "on-call team" consisting of but not limited to the following:

1. Cardiac surgeons
2. Cardiac anesthesiologist
3. Perfusionist
4. Hemodynamic monitoring technician
5. Circulating nurses × 2
6. Scrub nurse

After the team has been notified of a case, the response time of the team members should be 30 minutes or less.

Cardiac Surgery Policy: Team Notification of the Elective and Emergent Cardiac and Cardiothoracic Surgical Procedures

Cardiac surgery's policy is that the cardiac manager, or appointed designee, be responsible for mobilizing the cardiac team members for cardiac/cardiothoracic surgical procedures after notification from the referring surgeon.

The cardiac manager will notify the following:

1. Cardiac anesthesiologist
2. Perfusionist
3. Hemodynamic monitoring technician
4. Circulating nurses
5. Scrub nurse
6. Intensive care unit

Cardiac Surgery Nursing Procedure: Call Notification

Quality Outcome: Communication relating to the procedure, surgeon, patient, and time of surgery is relayed to the cardiac team in an effective manner.

Performed by: Cardiac manager

General Statement: The cardiac manager is responsible for communicating case information to the cardiac team and coordinating the team's activities in preparation for an elective or emergent cardiac surgical procedure.

Equipment: Organized list of team members' names, phone numbers, beeper numbers and cell phone numbers. Call schedule for anesthesia and perfusion.

Steps:	Rationale:
1. The cardiac manager is notified of the elective or emergent case from the surgery scheduling office or the surgeon.	One person is designated to adequately prepare the cardiac team, preventing confusion.
2. Procedure, diagnosis, patient name, age, surgeon and assistant, date, and time of surgery are communicated.	Pertinent patient information is received to prepare adequately for the impending surgery.
3. Cardiac manager notifies the perfusionist, anesthesiologist, and cardiac staff members by direct contact if during normal working hours or by telephone, beeper, or cell if after hours.	The team is mobilized and ready at the appropriate time.

Standard of Care: Cardiac Surgery: Staffing for Cardiac Surgical Procedures

I. Staffing for Cardiac Surgical Procedures
   A. Licensed personnel
      1. Cardiac surgeon
      2. Physician's assistant
      3. Cardiac anesthesiologist
      4. Perfusionist
      5. Hemodynamic monitoring specialist (may be licensed or nonlicensed)
      6. Two circulating nurses
      7. Scrub nurse (may be licensed or nonlicensed)
      8. Physician's assistant (optional)
   B. Nonlicensed personnel
      1. Scrub nurse
         a. ORT
      2. Hemodynamic monitoring specialist
         a. Anesthesia technician
         b. Cath lab technician
II. Educational Requirements for Cardiac Surgery
   A. Licensed personnel
      1. One year of general OR experience
      2. CPR certified
      3. ACLS certified
      4. CNOR preferred
      5. IABP certification (optional)
   B. Nonlicensed personnel
      1. One year of general OR experience
      2. EKG course
      3. CPR certification
III. Staffing Scheduling
   A. Regular time
      1. Flexible staffing hours to meet the needs of the case load
         a. Monday through Friday
   B. Call time to cover emergency cases and PTCA/atherectomy surgical support
      1. Rotated
         a. 24-hour coverage
            1. Weekends
            2. Holidays
         b. Evenings and nights, 5 days a week

IV. Call Notification
    A. Responsibility of the cardiac surgery manager
        1. Home phone
        2. Beeper or cell phone
    B. Response time of the team is 30 minutes

V. Clinical Indicators for Evaluation
    A. Team roles and responsibilities
    B. Staff accountability
    C. Productivity
    D. Staffing to meet the case load demands
    E. Availability of the staff on call
    F. Work attendance
    G. Continuing education

Standard of Care: Cardiac Surgery: Cardiac Team Networking

I. Team Building
   A. Goals
      1. Clarity in team goals
         a. Promotes commitment, recruitment, and retention
         b. Promotes loyalty
         c. Promotes productivity and positive patient outcomes
         d. "TEAM" Together Everyone Achieves More
      2. Improvement plan
         a. A system for meeting evolving surgeon and anesthesiologist needs and technology changes
         b. Versatility and flexibility
      3. Clearly defined roles
         a. Tap everyone's talent
      4. Clear communication
         a. Keep team members informed
         b. Listen actively
         c. Share information
         d. Network with other institutions and programs
      5. Beneficial team behaviors
         a. Encouragement of the team
      6. Well-defined procedure for decision making
         a. Database for change
         b. Consensus of opinion
         c. Empowerment
         d. Evidence-based practice
      7. Balanced participation
         a. Shared commitment
         b. Participation by all members
         c. Promote visibility
            1. Recognition
            2. Reinforcement of commitment and excitement
      8. Established ground rules
         a. Policies and procedures
         b. Regulatory compliance
         c. Standards of care
      9. Awareness of group process
         a. Stages to team development
            1. Orientation

    2. Adaptation
    3. Emergence
    4. Production
   b. Sensitivity to nonverbal communication
   c. Respect for others' views
  10. Use of the evidence-based approach
   a. Reliant data for problem solving
   b. Permanent solutions—not quick fixes

II. **Benefits of Teamwork**
 A. Quality
 B. Increased productivity
  1. A work environment that promotes, encourages, and supports
  2. Increased motivation
  3. Personnel accountability
 C. Versatility and flexibility
 D. The capability to problem solve effectively, and promote positive patient outcomes and customer satisfaction

III. **Teamwork Related to Cardiac Surgery**
 A. All licensed personnel working in the cardiac surgical suite can prepare and participate in the following but are not limited to
  1. Arterial line preparation
  2. Swan-Ganz line preparation
  3. Cell saver reservoir
  4. Patient assessment
  5. Patient positioning
  6. Assistant to the anesthesiologist
  7. Surgical prepping
  8. Intraoperative sponge, needle, and instrument counts
  9. Intraoperative documentation
  10. Preparation of the autotransfusion pleural drainage unit
 B. All nonlicensed personnel in the cardiac surgical suite can prepare and participate in the following but are not limited to
  1. Positioning of the noninvasive monitoring equipment
  2. The completion of the surgical counts with a licensed person
  3. CPR
 C. All circulating nurses and surgical techs can perform the second scrub role
  1. Conduit harvesting
  2. Femoral bypass preparation
  3. Heart holder
  4. The rinsing process associated with the implantation of a biological valve

- 5. Assistance with the placement of the intra-aortic balloon catheter
- 6. Staff relief for breaks/lunches

IV. Interdepartmental Networking
- A. Related departments
    1. Cardiac cath lab
    2. Intensive care unit
    3. Surgery
        - a. A.M. admissions
        - b. Patient units
    4. Cardiac step-down unit
    5. Emergency department
    6. Cardiology
    7. Diagnostic laboratory and blood bank
    8. Respiratory therapy
    9. Radiology
    10. Pharmacy
    11. Cardiac surgery office
    12. Anesthesia office

V. Benefits of Interdepartmental Networking
- A. Open communication between the units
    1. Strategic planning
        - a. Goals setting
        - b. Objectives reached
        - c. Continuity of patient care
        - d. Problem solving
        - e. Cost containment
        - f. Length of stay
- B. Standardization
    1. Standardization of supplies
    2. Standardization of equipment

VI. Networking with the Family
- A. Good communication
    1. Expectations
        - a. Time frame for surgery
        - b. Complications
            1. Cardiac supportive therapy
                - a. Presence of additional life support equipment that the family may be unaware of need for
        - c. Death
- B. Encouragement
- C. Support
    1. Clergy

    2. Advanced directives
    3. Ethics committee
 VII. Networking with the Cardiac Surgeon
   A. Case flow
   B. Supplies and instrumentation
   C. Standardization
   D. Mutual respect
   E. Commitment
 VIII. Clinical Indicator for Evaluation
   A. Evaluation of the cardiac surgery manager
   B. Productivity
   C. Case flow and time management
   D. Communication
   E. Personnel turnover rates
   F. Relationships with the related departments
    1. Effective problem solving
    2. Shared ideas
    3. Standardization
    4. Continuity of patient care

Education

chapter 3

Educational Program: Cardiac Surgery

The educational program devised for staffing the cardiac surgical suite involves basic educational requirements, a formal orientation process, and ongoing educational activities to evaluate methods of care for the cardiac surgical patient in an environment of changing technology.

The entry level for licensed personnel working in this environment includes current ACLS certification and at least 1 year of experience in general surgery. Nonlicensed personnel, ORTS, must have a minimum of 1 year of experience in general surgery, successful completion of an EKG course, and current CPR certification.

Each orientee is given an introduction to the cardiac surgical team and his or her roles, philosophy of cardiac surgery, a history of cardiac surgical procedures performed with the anticipated case volume, and a tour of the cardiac surgical suite. A cardiac surgery orientation manual is made available as a reference guide for the orientee. This manual includes the goals, objectives, and expectations of the orientee, standards of care, special cardiac surgical procedures, and an introduction to the special equipment necessary for cardiac surgical cases.

The orientation process is structured for each individual job role and involves the use of an experience preceptor. The preceptor is an advanced clinical nurse with a minimum of 2 years of experience in cardiac surgical nursing who demonstrates proficiency in all aspects of cardiac surgical nursing, both the scrub and circulating roles. The preceptor applies the nursing process, integrating scientific principles and technological knowledge to all aspects of care for the patient undergoing cardiac surgery. This individual must demonstrate accountability, responsibility, and leadership skills; show interest in teaching; and maintain good interdepartmental working relationships.

The preceptor is responsible for coordinating the orientee's daily assignment, incorporating the necessary cardiac surgical experience to facilitate the transition of the orientee to cardiac surgical nursing.

The preceptor uses formal skills competency checklists as tools to evaluate the orientee on a weekly basis. The preceptor reports to the cardiac surgery manager regarding the level of performance of the orientee and continued educational needs. The time frame of the orientation process is determined by the job role, previous experience of the orientee, case volume and exposure to the different cardiac surgical procedures, and progress of the orientee.

Integration of the cardiac surgical policy and procedures is critical to the education process.

At the end of the orientation process, the orientee has an opportunity to evaluate the effectiveness of the preceptor.

The cardiac team members meet on a monthly basis to discuss goals and evaluate methods of care for the cardiac surgical patient. Shared goals are established to promote commitment, loyalty, and productivity.

Teamwork is emphasized. The benefits of teamwork permit continuity of care with the capability to problem solve more efficiently, provide increased motivation of the team members, promote personnel accountability, and build avenues for versatility and flexibility, adding increased quality to the services provided.

Continuing education of new equipment or changes in technology is also provided. The team is challenged and encouraged to participate with the topic selection. Networking with other institutions regarding cardiac surgery is encouraged.

Cardiac Surgery: Policy: Educational Requirements, Licensed Cardiac Nursing Staff

Cardiac surgery's policy is to standardize the level of entry practice required by the licensed nursing staff working within the cardiac surgical suite. The following criteria must be met but are not limited to

1. Minimum of 1 year of general surgery experience
2. Current CPR certification
3. Current ACLS certification

The staff is trained and prepared to meet the needs of the critically ill cardiac patient and to intervene and perform with the highest level of expertise with cardiac life support.

Cardiac Surgery: Policy: Educational Requirements, Nonlicensed Cardiac Nursing Staff

Cardiac surgery's policy is to standardize the level of entry practice required by the nonlicensed nursing staff working within the cardiac surgical suite. The following criteria must be met but the criteria are not limited to

1. Minimum of 1 year of general surgery experience
2. Current CPR certification
3. Successful completion of an EKG course

The staff is trained and prepared to meet the needs of the critically ill cardiac patient and to intervene and perform with the highest level of expertise with cardiac life support.

Standard of Care: Cardiac Surgery: Cardiac Surgery Orientation

I. Introduction to the Surgical Team
   A. Introduction to the team members
      1. Individual team roles and responsibilities
      2. Coordinated team effort
         a. Overlapping job responsibilities
         b. Cross training
   B. History of cardiac surgery
      1. Types of cardiac surgical procedures performed
      2. Case load
   C. Tour of the cardiac surgical suite
      1. Location of supplies, equipment, and instrumentation
         a. Locator file for quick reference
      2. Surgeon's preference cards
      3. Standard equipment used during a cardiac surgical procedure
      4. Emergency drugs
   D. Philosophy of cardiac surgery
      1. Quality patient care
      2. Cost containment
   E. Networking with the cardiac-related units

II. The Orientation Process
   A. Orientation manual
      1. Goals
      2. Objectives
      3. Expectations
      4. Standards of care
      5. Special cardiac surgical procedures
      6. Special equipment
   B. Preceptor program
      1. Orientation objectives
      2. Job description
      3. Time frame for the orientation process
      4. Weekly orientation progress report
      5. Orientation evaluation
      6. Evaluation of the preceptor
      7. Basic technical competency checkoff list
         a. Scrub role
            1. First scrub role
            2. Second scrub role
         b. Circulating role

III. Role of the Preceptor
   A. Coordinate of the orientee's assignment on a daily basis
   B. Incorporate the necessary cardiac surgical experience for the orientee
   C. Share with the cardiac manager the level of performance of an assignment of the orientee and continued learning needs
   D. Facilitate the transition of the orientee to cardiac surgical nursing
IV. Criteria for the Preceptor
   A. Advanced clinical nurse
      1. Technical knowledge of cardiac surgical nursing, minimum of 2 years
         a. Demonstrates proficiency in all aspects of cardiac surgical nursing
            1. Circulating role
            2. Scrub role
   B. Application of the nursing process for the care of a patient undergoing the cardiac surgical experience
      1. Relates scientific principles and technological knowledge to all aspects of cardiac surgical nursing.
   C. Demonstrates accountability and responsibility
   D. Demonstrates leadership qualities
   E. Maintains appropriate interdepartmental working relationships
   F. Demonstrates an interest in teaching
V. Education
   A. Licensed staff
      1. CPR certified
      2. ACLS certified
   B. Surgical technicians
      1. CPR certified
      2. Completion of an EKG course
   C. Utilization of the nursing process
      1. Assessment
      2. Planning
      3. Implementing
      4. Evaluating the response
   D. Continuing education
      1. Monthly cardiac inservice meetings
         a. Encourage professional growth
         b. Enhance the knowledge of cardiac surgical nursing
         c. Relevant continuing education programs
            1. Cardiac procedures
            2. New technology

                3. Infection control
                4. Safety
        E. Support research
            1. Raise the quality of patient care
            2. Initiate change
VI. Ongoing Competency Review
    A. Maintenance of current licensure
        1. Nursing license
        2. ACLS certification
        3. CPR certification
    B. Annual assessment evaluation based on the job description
        1. Supervisor observation
        2. Peer review
        3. Pay for performance
VII. Clinical Indicators for Evaluation
    A. Educational prerequisites
    B. Length of the orientation process
    C. Preceptor
    D. Performance of the individual
    E. Utilization of the nursing process
    F. Completion of the skills checklist
    G. Pertinent continuing education

Proficiency Skills Checklist: Circulating Nurse

I. Goals
   A. Development of professional culture with a sound knowledge base in cardiac surgical procedures
      1. Autonomy
      2. Accountability
      3. Creativity
      4. Expert practice
         a. Prioritizing actions to meet the changing status of the patient
         b. Versatility
   B. Quality
      1. Continuous improvement
         a. Systems of cardiac surgical care
         b. Process of patient care delivery
   C. Networking
      1. Development of a collaborative partnership
         a. Medical staff
         b. Team members
         c. Cardiac units
   D. Financial
      1. Cost containment
II. General Competency
   A. General OR nursing experience
      1. Circulating role
      2. Scrub role
   B. CPR certification
   C. ACLS certification
   D. Knowledge of the anatomy and physiology of the heart
III. Knowledge Demonstrated During the Preoperative Phase
   A. Preparation of the room and equipment
      1. Room and equipment prepared based on the individual patient needs and the type of procedure
      2. Acquisition of the pertinent supplies and equipment
         a. CABG procedures
         b. Valve replacement/repair procedures
         c. Cardiothoracic procedures
      3. Checking and testing the equipment
      4. Opening case supplies
      5. Fluid line preparation

        a. Invasive line preparation
        b. Cardiosupportive drug therapy
            1. Names of the cardiosupportive drugs
            2. Uses/contraindications/abnormal reactions
            3. Usual dose
            4. Delivery system
            5. How the drug is supplied
    B. Assessment of the patient
        1. Proper identification
        2. Chart review
            a. Interpret abnormal laboratory tests
        3. Nursing assessment
        4. Surgical shave prep
        5. Patient education
    C. Safe transport of the patient to the surgical suite
IV. Knowledge Demonstrated Intraoperatively
    A. Placement of the noninvasive monitoring equipment
    B. Assistance with invasive line placement
    C. Interpretation of electrocardiographic information
        1. Recognition of dysrhythmias
        2. Treatment modalities for dysrhythmias
            a. Drug therapy
            b. Pacing therapy
            c. Ablation therapy
                1. Temporary pacing wires
                      a. Alligator clips
                      b. Temporary electrodes
                2. Permanent pacing electrodes
            d. Initiate CPR
            e. Defibrillate, as appropriate
                1. Joule settings for internal and external defibrillation
                2. Synchronized or unsynchronized
                3. Administer routinely used emergency drugs
    D. Interpretation of hemodynamic parameters
        1. CVP
        2. Arterial pressures
        3. Cardiac output
        4. SVR
        5. Pulmonary artery pressures
        6. Pulmonary capillary wedge pressures
        7. Mixed venous saturation
        8. Cardiac index

Proficiency Skills Checklist: Circulating Nurse

E. Administer fluid/blood/blood components
F. Patient safety
 1. Positioning
    a. CABG procedures
    b. Valve replacement/repair procedures
    c. Cardiothoracic procedures
       1. Supine approach
       2. Thoracic approach
 2. Electrocautery safety
 3. Infection control
 4. Surgical skin preps
    a. CABG procedures
    b. Valve procedures
    c. Cardiothoracic procedures
 5. Surgical counts
    a. Sponges
    b. Instruments
    c. Suture
G. Risk management
 1. Environmental conditions
 2. Universal precautions
 3. Infection control
 4. Variance reporting
 5. Perioperative documentation
H. Coordination of the multidisciplined team
 1. Needs of the surgeon
 2. Needs of the anesthesiologist
 3. Needs of the perfusionist
 4. Needs of the hemodynamic monitoring specialist
 5. Needs of the scrub nurse/tech
I. Special procedure needs
 1. VADS
 2. IABP
 3. Automatic internal cardioverter defibrillator
 4. Femoral cannulation
 5. IMA harvesting
 6. Cell saver
 7. Autotransfusion pleural drainage unit
 8. Transesophageal echocardiography
 9. Handling of implants
 10. Documentation of implants
 11. Cardiopulmonary bypass

    a. Aorta—right atrium
    b. Femoral artery—right atrium
    c. Femoral artery—femoral vein
    d. Reimplementation of cardiopulmonary bypass
  J. Anticoagulation process
  K. Myocardial protection techniques
    1. Warm continuous
    2. Cold intermittent
  L. Standards of care
    1. CABG
    2. Valve replacement/repair
    3. Cardiothoracic
  M. Use of the nursing process
    1. Assessment
    2. Planning
    3. Implementing
    4. Evaluating
  N. Critical thinking
    1. Prioritizing actions in an emergent situation
V. Knowledge Demonstrated Postoperatively
  A. Safe transfer of the patient to the unit
    1. Transfer of invasive lines to the transport monitor
    2. Transfer of the patient from the surgical bed to the intensive care unit bed
    3. Report given to the intensive care nurse
  B. Surgical suite cleanup
    1. Restocking of the supplies and equipment

Standard of Care: Cardiac Surgery: Proficiency Skills Checklist: Scrub Nurse

I. Goals
   A. Development of professional culture with a sound knowledge base in cardiac surgical procedures
      1. Autonomy
      2. Accountability
      3. Creativity
      4. Expert practice
         a. Prioritizing actions to meet the changing status of the patient
         b. Versatility
   B. Quality
      1. Continuous improvement
         a. Systems of cardiac surgical care
         b. Process of patient care delivery
         c. Patients' length of stay and outcomes
   C. Networking
      1. Development of a collaborative partnership
         a. Medical staff
         b. Team members
   D. Financial
      1. Cost containment
II. General Competency
   A. General OR nursing experience
      1. Licensed scrub
         a. Circulating role
      2. Surgical tech
   B. Education
      1. Licensed scrub
         a. CPR certification
         b. ACLS certification
      2. Surgical tech scrub
         a. CPR certification
         b. Basic EKG course
   C. Knowledge of the anatomy and physiology of the heart
   D. Knowledge of the heart–lung machine
      1. Function
      2. Dynamics
      3. Extracorporeal circuits
III. Knowledge Demonstrated During the Preoperative Phase

A. Preparation of the room and equipment
 1. Room and equipment prepared based on the individual patient needs and the type of procedure
 2. Acquisition of the pertinent supplies and equipment
    a. CABG procedures
    b. Valve replacement/repair procedures
    c. Cardiothoracic procedures
 3. Assessing the case supplies for sterility
    a. Opening case supplies
B. Sterile field preparation
 1. Instruments organized effectively for the following:
    a. CABG procedures
 2. Vein/radial artery harvesting procedure
 3. IMA harvesting procedure
    a. Valve replacement/repair procedures
 4. Handling the graft
 5. Handling of the annuloplasty ring
 6. Special sutures
    a. Cardiothoracic procedures
 7. Instruments appropriate for the surgical approach used
    a. Supine approach
    b. Posteriolateral thoracotomy approach
    c. Handling grafts and conduits

IV. Knowledge Demonstrated Intraoperatively
  A. Interpretation of electrocardiographic information
   1. Recognition of dysrhythmias
   2. Treatment modalities for dysrhythmias
      a. Drug therapy
      b. Pacing therapy
      c. Ablation therapy
         1. Temporary pacing wires
            a. Alligator clips
            b. Temporary electrodes
         2. Permanent pacing electrodes
            a. Initiate CPR
  B. Interpretation of hemodynamic parameters
   1. CVP
   2. Arterial pressures
   3. Pulmonary artery pressures
   4. Pulmonary capillary wedge pressures
   5. Cardiac output
  C. Draping procedure

Standard of Care: Cardiac Surgery: Proficiency Skills Checklist: Scrub Nurse

        1. CABG procedures
        2. Valve procedures
        3. Cardiothoracic procedures
           a. Supine approach
           b. Thoracic approach
   D. Patient safety
        1. Electrocautery and fire safety
        2. Infection control
        3. Surgical counts
           a. Sponges
           b. Instruments
           c. Suture
   E. Cardiopulmonary bypass
        1. Preparation of the extracorporeal table circuits
        2. Special perfusion cannulas
        3. Procedures for implementing cardiopulmonary bypass
           a. Aorta—right atrium
           b. Femoral artery—right atrium
           c. Femoral artery—femoral vein
               1. Electively
               2. Emergently
               3. Reimplementation
           d. Anticoagulation process
               1. Ensuring that heparin was given prebypass
               2. Use of the cell saver and cardiotomy aspirating circuits
           e. Cannulation process
               1. Pursestring sutures
               2. Extracorporeal circuit connections
           f. Decannulation process
           g. Reimplementation process for cardiopulmonary bypass
   F. Myocardial protection techniques
        1. Warm continuous
        2. Cold intermittent
           a. Appropriate time of reversal
   G. Comprehension of the procedure to be performed
        1. Sequence of events
           a. CABG procedure
           b. Valve replacement/repair procedure
           c. Cardiothoracic procedure
               1. Ascending aortic repairs
               2. Descending aortic repairs
        2. Surgeon's preferences and routine

    H. Risk management
        1. Environmental conditions
        2. Universal precautions
        3. Infection control
        4. Variance reporting
    I. Communication with the multidiscipled team
        1. Needs of the surgeon
        2. Needs of the perfusionist
        3. Needs of the patient
        4. Assistance from the circulating nurse
    J. Special procedure needs
        1. VADS
        2. IABP
        3. Automatic internal cardioverter defibrillator
        4. Femoral cannulation
        5. IMA harvesting
        6. Cell saver
        7. Autotransfusion pleural drainage unit
        8. Transesophageal echocardiography
        9. Handling of implants and conduits
    K. Standards of care
        1. CABG
        2. Valve replacement/repair
        3. Cardiothoracic
    L. Use of the nursing process
        1. Assessment
        2. Planning
        3. Implementing
        4. Evaluating
    M. Critical thinking
        1. Prioritizing actions in an emergent situation
V. Knowledge Demonstrated Postoperatively
    A. Care and handling of the instrumentation
    B. Appropriate hazardous waste procedure
    C. Surgical suite cleanup
        1. Restocking of the supplies and equipment

Cardiac Surgery: Policy: Monthly Cardiac Inservice Meetings

Cardiac surgery's policy is that monthly staff inservices be scheduled with time dedicated to the following but not limited to

1. Cardiac surgical procedures
2. New equipment
3. Staff concerns
4. Safety

The dates, times, meeting agendas, and team members present are documented.

Cardiac Surgery: Nursing Procedure: Monthly Cardiac Inservice Meetings

Quality Outcome: The cardiac team meets on a routine basis to discuss goals, assists members of the team, and evaluates methods of care for the cardiac surgical patient.
Performed by: Cardiac team members/cardiac surgery manager
General Statement: A monthly meeting is established by the cardiac manager and held for the cardiac surgical team members.
Equipment: Not applicable

Steps:	Rationale:
1. The cardiac manager designates a meeting time to be held monthly that will allow all members of the cardiac surgical team to be present.	A routine is established for monthly cardiac staff meetings incorporating all team members.
2. Before the meeting, the cardiac manager prepares an agenda that is presented to the team along with notification of the time, date, and location of the meeting.	Written documentation of the upcoming meeting helps the team prepare their time appropriately.
3. The team members are asked to sign in on a sheet of paper designating the cardiac staff meetings.	An attendance record is kept for future reference.
4. Any new procedure, instrumentation, or equipment is discussed. Staff concerns or questions are shared and answered.	These meetings provide support of team members' roles and evaluate methods of care for the cardiac surgical patient.
5. A log is kept of the cardiac meetings, attendance, and agendas.	It follows JCAHO and government regulations.

Scheduling

chapter 4

It is the cardiac surgery policy that all patients requiring cardiac surgical procedures be scheduled with the hospital's admission's office, the surgery office, and the cardiac surgery manager to facilitate the following:

1. Reserved hospital bed on the appropriate unit at the designated time
2. Availability of the cardiac surgical suite
3. Appropriate communication to the cardiac team

Cardiac Surgery: Nursing Procedure: Scheduling of the Elective Cardiac Surgical Procedure

Quality Outcome: The cardiac team is available and prepared for the cardiac surgical patient.
Performed by: Unit secretary and cardiac surgery office
General Statement: The following pertinent scheduling information is received and documented:

A. Patient's name, age, address, and telephone number
B. Diagnosis and procedure
   1. If CABG, type of vascular conduits
      a. Saphenous veins
      b. Internal mammary artery(s)
      c. Cephalic veins
      d. Radial artery
      e. Synthetic grafts
   2. If valve procedure
      a. Valve position: aortic, mitral, or tricuspid
      b. Repair or replacement
      c. Type of valve: mechanical or biological
      d. Need for intraoperative transesophageal echocardiography
   3. If cardiothoracic procedure
      a. Position: left or right lateral
      b. Cardiopulmonary bypass route: aorta-right atrial cannulation, femoral-femoral cannulation, or femoral artery-right atrial cannulation
C. Date and time of surgery
D. Admission mode: prehospitalized or same-day admission
E. Primary and assisting surgeons
F. Special needs of the patient/physician or additional equipment requests
G. Initial cardiac surgical procedure versus previous cardiac surgical procedure
   1. Type of previous cardiac surgery
      a. If CABG
         1. Location of patent grafts
         2. Availability of graft conduits
      b. If valve procedure
         1. Median sternotomy approach versus the thoracotomy approach

Equipment: Not applicable

Steps:	Rationale:
1. The unit secretary receives booking information.	Case information is documented in the surgery scheduling book or electronic scheduling module, including date, time, and person who took the booking.
2. The unit secretary contacts the cardiac manager, and case scheduling information is relayed.	The cardiac manager informs the cardiac team of the procedure, date and time, surgeons, and any special requests. The team is prepared for the surgical procedure.
3. The case is placed on the written surgery schedule and distributed to the appropriate units.	Communication is facilitated to the units providing patient care and aids in planning for appropriate staff mix.

Standard of Care: Cardiac Surgery: Scheduling of the Cardiac Surgical Procedures

I. Patient Is Scheduled for Cardiac Surgery with the Surgery Department and Cardiac Surgery Manager
   A. Electively
      1. Same-day admission, whenever a patient's condition permits
      2. As soon as the surgery schedule permits
   B. Emergently
      1. Transferred from the emergency department
         a. Cardiothoracic trauma
         b. Ascending aortic aneurysm
         c. Thoracic aneurysm
      2. Received directly from the catheterization laboratory
         a. Unstable angina
         b. Left main coronary artery occlusion
         c. Failed PTCA, coronary stenting
         d. Papillary muscle rupture
      3. Received directly from the intensive care unit
         a. Re-exploration of the mediastinum for hemorrhage

II. Scheduling for Cardiac Surgical Backup Support
   A. PTCA coverage
   B. Coronary atherectomy/stenting

III. Scheduling Information
   A. Pertinent patient history
      1. Patient's name, address, age, and telephone number
      2. Diagnosis and procedure
     If valve procedure
         a. Valve position: aortic, mitral, or tricuspid
         b. Repair or replacement
         c. Type of valve: mechanical or biological
         d. Need for intraoperative transesophageal echocardiography
     If CABG procedure
         a. Type of vascular conduits
            1. Saphenous veins
            2. Cephalic veins
            3. Internal mammary artery(s)
            4. Radial artery(s)
            5. Synthetic grafts

        If cardiothoracic procedure
- a. Surgical position: left lateral or right lateral
- b. Cardiopulmonary bypass route
  1. Aorta-right atrial cannulation
  2. Femoral-femoral cannulation
  3. Femoral artery-right atrial cannulation

        If PTCA/coronary atherectomy/stenting
- a. Team notification
- b. All members present for the duration of the procedure, if requested
  1. Date and time of surgical procedure
  2. Current condition of the patient

B. Mode of admission to the surgical unit
C. Name of surgeon and assistants
D. Any special surgeon or patient needs
E. Date and time procedure is booked
F. Name of staff receiving the scheduling information
G. Special equipment requested
H. Initial cardiac procedure versus previous cardiac surgery
1. Type of cardiac procedure performed in the past
   a. If CABG surgery, patent grafts, their location, and current availability of graft sites
   b. If valve surgery, median sternotomy versus a thoracotomy incision site

IV. Clinical Indicators for Evaluation of Scheduling Effectiveness
A. Data collection at periodic intervals for review
1. Variation between actual number of cases and those that were predicted
2. Operating hours available versus the actual hours used due to
   a. Variations in the schedule
   b. Noncompliance with protocols
3. Monitoring average surgical time
   a. Preparation time
   b. Cleanup time
   c. Turnover time
4. Instrument/equipment availability related to scheduling

Cardiac Surgery: Nursing Procedure: Scheduling the Emergent Cardiac Surgical Procedure

Quality Outcome: The cardiac surgical team is mobilized quickly and efficiently to meet the needs of the critical cardiac patient.

Performed by: Cardiac manager or cardiac surgeon

General Statement: The surgeon notifies the cardiac manager of an emergent case. The cardiac manager then notifies the team members, relaying the following pertinent information to facilitate the surgical process:

1. Patient's diagnosis, current physical status, sense of urgency
2. Name of anesthesiologist, surgeon, and procedure
3. Any special needs of the patient, surgeon, or additional equipment needs

The required team response is 30 minutes.

Equipment: Call notification list consisting of team members' home, cell, and pager numbers

Steps:	Rationale:
1. The surgeon communicates the emergent need to the cardiac manager. The location of the patient is verified, along with the estimated time of surgery.	Communication is facilitated when one team member is in charge of team mobilization.
2. The cardiac manager mobilizes the team. The procedure, the name of the operating surgeon, and the immediate physical status of the patient are relayed.	Facilitates the preoperative preparation and the perioperative plan of care.
3. The cardiac manager notifies the intensive care unit of the impending case and estimated arrival time to the unit with the patient.	The unit has a bed and staff available for the postoperative cardiac patient.

Steps:	Rationale:
4. The OR suite is prepared to meet the needs of the patient, surgeon, and procedure.	Emergency equipment is available and is ready for use.
5. The patient is brought to the cardiac OR suite as soon as all team members are present.	The cardiac team is prepared.

Nursing Procedure: Scheduling the Emergent Cardiac Surgical Procedure

Cardiac Surgery: Nursing Procedure: Same-Day Admission of the Cardiac Surgical Patient

Quality Outcome: The length of stay is shortened by admitting the patient the morning of surgery.

Performed by: Admission nurse or cardiac office coordinator

General Statement: Cardiac patients electively scheduled for cardiac surgery can be admitted the morning of surgery. All preoperative labs are drawn on an outpatient basis. The completed chart consisting of consents, lab results, history and physical, preoperative orders, and the preoperative nursing physical assessment are organized the afternoon before the scheduled procedure. Lab results are screened for abnormalities, and the surgeon is notified.

Equipment: Organized chart containing the following:

Appropriate consents
Preoperative physical assessment
History and physical
Recorded lab results
Preoperative orders

Steps:	Rationale:
1. The admission and surgery offices are notified of the patient's name, age, address and phone, the type of surgical procedure, the date and time that the procedure is to be performed, the name of the surgeon to initiate the surgical process and assistants, and the name of the insurance carrier if applicable.	Information regarding the patient and the surgical procedure is documented. The admissions office is responsible for bed control.
2. The cardiac manager is notified of the scheduled case and notifies the team members.	The cardiac team members are prepared to meet the needs of the surgeon and the patient at the appropriate time.
3. The patient and family receive preoperative education, including resource literature.	The patient and family receive detailed information regarding the disease process, surgical plan, and postoperative expectations.

Steps:	Rationale:
4. Lab work is completed before surgery.	Lab is drawn before the scheduled surgery to prevent delays. Type and cross-match for blood or designated donor blood must be completed within 48 to 72 hours of the scheduled procedure.
5. The chart is complete the afternoon before the surgical procedure, history and physical present, appropriate consents signed and witnessed, lab results documented, and preoperative orders are written.	Lab work is screened for any abnormalities, and the surgeon notified, preventing surgical delays.
6. The patient arrives in the AM surgical admission area 1.5 hours before the scheduled surgery time.	This allows adequate time to prepare the patient for surgery.
7. The preoperative physical assessment is completed.	The patient's physical condition is evaluated to facilitate and individualize perioperative care.
8. The preoperative shave prep is completed using a hair clipper.	Shaving should be done as close to the operative procedure as possible. Microscopic abrasions can occur during the hair removal process, providing a good culture medium for microorganisms with subsequent risk of wound infection.
9. Preoperative medications are given if ordered.	Preoperative narcotics relieve anxiety related to the surgical procedure. Prophylactic antibiotics may be given.
10. The circulating nurse identifies the patient, verifies the surgical procedure and operating surgeon, and completes the operative checklist. Patient questions are answered.	The patient's identity is confirmed. Phases and expectations of the preoperative period are explained, decreasing patient anxiety.

Nursing Procedure: Same-Day Admission of the Cardiac Surgical Patient

Steps:

11. The circulating nurse transports the patient to the OR suite 45 minutes before the scheduled surgery time. The patient is positioned supine on the surgical table. Noninvasive monitors are applied.

Rationale:

This permits time for invasive line placement and intubation by the anesthesiologist in preparation for cardiac surgical intervention.

Standard of Care: Cardiac Surgery: Same-Day Admissions of the Cardiac Surgical Patient

I. Prerequisites for Same-Day Admissions
   A. Stable patient
   B. Lab work drawn on an outpatient basis up to 2 weeks before the surgical procedure
   C. Type and cross-match for blood are completed within 48–72 hours of the surgical procedure. Designated donor blood is prepared on request.
   D. Patient and family education
      1. Disease process
      2. Surgical plan
      3. Postoperative expectations
   E. Surgical consents signed and witnessed
      1. Surgical procedure consent
      2. Anesthesia consent (if applicable)
      3. Blood transfusion consent form
   F. Pertinent patient information organized in a chart the afternoon before surgery
      1. Lab results are documented.
         a. The surgeon is notified of any abnormalities.
      2. History and physical
      3. Nursing physical assessment
      4. Surgical consents
      5. Preoperative physician orders

II. Morning of Admission
   A. Arrives at the surgery holding area 1.5 hours before the scheduled surgical time
   B. NPO past midnight before the morning of the surgical procedure
   C. The surgery admission nurse properly identifies the patient.
      1. An identification band is placed on the patient's wrist.
      2. Blood-processing identification band is placed on the patient's wrist.
      3. An allergy alert band is placed on the patient's wrist, if applicable.
   D. The patient is dressed in a hospital gown.
   E. All jewelry is removed.
   F. All prostheses are removed
      1. Glasses, contact lenses
      2. Hearing aids
      3. Dentures (dependent on anesthesia request)

a. All personal effects are left with the family.
 G. Preoperative nursing physical assessment
  1. Color of the skin
  2. The patient's ability to respond appropriately
   a. Level of consciousness
  3. Respiratory assessment
  4. Presence of pain
   a. Type
   b. Location
   c. Duration
   d. Intensity
  5. Vital signs, completed and recorded
  6. Emotional status
  7. Any condition that may dispose the patient to infection
  8. Any sensory or motor impairments
 H. Formulation of nursing care plan to achieve patient's needs and set priorities for goals that will meet expected outcomes.
 I. The circulating nurse answers any patient questions regarding the surgical procedure.
 J. The preoperative shave prep is done per physician's order and case-specific cardiac shave protocol.
 K. Preoperative medication given
  1. Narcotics
  2. Antibiotics
 L. The surgical documentation records are identified with the patient's name.
 M. The preoperative surgical checklist is completed and signed.
III. Transfer of the Patient to the Surgical Suite
 A. The circulating nurse introduces himself or herself to the patient.
  1. The circulating nurse requests the patient to acknowledge his or her own name and birth date, the name of the primary surgeon, and the type of procedure.
  2. The circulating nurse verifies the NPO status.
  3. The chart is checked for completeness.
  4. The nursing physical assessment is completed.
  5. Any patient or family questions are answered.
 B. The circulating nurse documents the time the patient is taken to the surgical suite.
  1. Requests additional assistance, if needed, to transport the patient safely to the surgical suite
 C. The patient is positioned on the surgical table according to the procedure to be performed.

      D. Noninvasive monitoring equipment is applied to the patient for hemodynamic monitoring perioperatively.
IV. Clinical Indicators for Evaluation
    A. Data collection
        1. Documentation of variances
           a. Patient
           b. Surgery time: actual start time versus time that surgery was scheduled
           c. Lab results
           d. Expected outcomes versus actual outcomes
        2. Patient comprehension and education
           a. Communication with the family

Cardiac Surgery: Policy: Scheduling Cardiac Surgical Support for Percutaneous Transluminal Coronary Angioplasty, Coronary Atherectomy, or Coronary Stenting Procedures

It is cardiac surgery policy that patients undergoing percutaneous transluminal coronary angioplasty, coronary atherectomy, or coronary stenting procedures that require cardiac surgical team backup be scheduled with the surgery office and the cardiac surgery manager to facilitate the following:

1. The availability of the cardiac surgical suite
2. The appropriate communication and coordination of the cardiac surgical team

Cardiac Surgery Policy and Nursing Procedure: PTCA, Coronary Atherectomy, and Coronary Stenting Surgical Standby Support

Quality Outcome: The cardiac team and the surgical suite are prepared to receive a patient emergently from the cath lab should the need arise.

Performed by:

Cardiac anesthesiologist
Perfusionist
Circulating nurses
Hemodynamic monitoring specialist
Scrub nurse

General Statement: The cardiac manager coordinates the notification of the cardiac team for the stand-by coverage. The cardiac team is required to be present in the hospital, dressed in scrubs, and ready to operate should the need arise. The team is available until the "clear" sign is received from the cath lab.

Equipment:

Cardiac case cart of supplies
Perfusion supplies
Emergency equipment

Steps:	Rationale:

1. The cardiac manager notifies the cardiac team of the stand-by coverage. The cardiac manager relays the pertinent patient information to the team, including, but not limited to,
  a. Physical condition of the patient
  b. Vessels or grafts to be dilated
  c. Location of the obstruction
	The entire team is gathered for the stand-by coverage in case the patient requires emergency coronary artery bypass surgery. The pertinent patient information facilitates the intraoperative plan of care.

2. The team response is 30 minutes. The team changes from street clothes to scrub clothes.	The team is dressed in scrubs to facilitate the surgical suite preparation. Time is life.

Steps:	Rationale:
3. The circulating and scrub nurses spread the cardiac case supplies around the surgical suite. The surgical suite is assessed for the correct equipment.	Organizing the supplies and instruments will save valuable time needed later.
4. The hemodynamic monitoring specialist ensures that the monitoring equipment is available.	The room is prepared for an emergency procedure.
5. The perfusionist ensures that the perfusion equipment is near the heart–lung machine.	The room is prepared for an emergency procedure.
6. The instruments and supplies are not opened unless the patient has to come to surgery.	Supplies are not wasted.
7. The cardiac team remains in the surgery department until the clear sign has been received from the cath lab.	The team remains until the patient is safely through the procedure.

Standard of Care: Cardiac Surgery: Percutaneous Transluminal Coronary Angioplasty, Coronary Atherectomy, or Coronary Stenting Surgical Stand-By Support

I. Scheduling
   A. The procedure is scheduled with the surgery office and cardiac surgery manager.
      1. Date and time of surgical backup support needed
      2. Cardiologist performing the procedure
      3. Risk or rating of the procedure
      4. Coronary arteries involved
         a. Single vessel
         b. Multiple vessels
         c. Vein grafts
   B. Availability of the designated surgical suite is confirmed.
   C. The cardiac team members are notified.
      1. Date and time of procedure
      2. Any special patient considerations
         a. Dilation of vein grafts
II. Team Responsibilities During the PTCA/Coronary Atherectomy/Coronary Stenting Coverage
   A. All team members are present during the entire procedure until the clear sign is received from the cardiac catheterization lab.
   B. The cardiac surgical suite is prepared for the possibility of an emergent revascularization procedure.
      1. The supplies and instruments needed for a CABG procedure are in the cardiac surgical suite.
         a. The case supplies are not opened until the team is given notification that the patient requires emergency surgery.
         b. The supplies are organized so that they can be opened quickly.
      2. Perfusion supplies are available, but not opened.
         a. The perfusion circuit for cardiopulmonary bypass is not set up until the team is given notification that the patient requires emergency surgery.
      3. All equipment is available, inspected, and connected to power sources.
III. Patients Requiring Emergent Cardiac Surgical Revascularization
   A. Surgery notification from the catheterization lab

1. Condition of patient
   a. Stable
   b. Unstable
2. Arrival time of the patient to surgery
3. Invasive lines present and their location
   a. Arterial line
   b. Swan-Ganz catheter
   c. Foley catheter
   d. Coronary perfusion catheter
   e. Pacing catheters
4. Cardiac supportive drug therapy instituted
   a. Type of drug
   b. Drug dose
   c. Rate of infusion
5. Mechanical assist devices present
   a. Ventilator/ambu bag
   b. Intra-aortic balloon
   c. CPR in progress
6. Special patient considerations
   a. Allergies
   b. Patient refusal of blood or blood products
   c. Fear
   d. Pain
   e. Implanted devices
   f. External implants/prosthesis
7. Blood availability
   a. Blood typed and cross-matched

B. Facilitation of surgical intervention, intraoperative priorities
   1. Quick nursing physical assessment
      a. The perioperative plan of care is reassessed as changes in the patient's hemodynamic status occur.
   2. Surgical positioning of the patient
   3. Noninvasive monitoring equipment is applied while invasive lines are being inserted.
   4. Emotional support is provided.
   5. Temperature control is supported with the use of extra blankets, as needed.
   6. Pain control is provided.
   7. Surgical shave prep is completed.
   8. Dispersive electrode pads are positioned.
   9. Surgical prep is initiated.
   10. Surgeons are scrubbed.

IV. Special Considerations
   A. Expedite the initiation of cardiopulmonary bypass
      1. If CPR is in progress
         a. CPR is not interrupted until cardiopulmonary bypass is initiated or the patient is successfully resuscitated.
      2. Cardiopulmonary bypass may be initiated through the femoral artery and vein.
         a. The femoral cannulation tray is available.
         b. Femoral arterial and venous perfusion cannulas are available.
   B. Anticipation of additional cardiac supportive drugs
      1. Epinephrine
      2. Levophed
      3. Lidocaine
      4. Dopamine
   C. Anticipation of hemodynamic supportive devices
      1. Intra-aortic balloon pump
      2. Atrial-ventricular pacing wires and generator
      3. LVAD/RVAD
   D. Communication with the family and the intensive care unit
      1. Progress/status of the patient
      2. The estimated time of transfer to the intensive care unit
         a. Verbal and documented patient transfer report
      3. Intraoperative mortality

V. Quality Indicators for Evaluation
   A. Effective communication between the catheterization lab and cardiac surgery
   B. Team response to surgical backup notification
   C. Expedient surgical case preparation
   D. Alternative plans of care to meet the changing hemodynamic needs of the critical patient
   E. Patient outcome
      1. Safety
      2. Infection control
      3. Hemodynamic status

Standard of Care: Cardiac Surgery: Repeat Cardiac Surgical Procedures

I. Preliminary Case Preparation
   A. Scheduling
      1. Is it indicated on the surgery schedule as "reoperation"?
      2. The cardiac manager relates case information to the cardiac team.
      3. The history of previous cardiac surgery is acquired.
         a. If previous CABG
            1. The location of any patent grafts
            2. Harvesting sites available for coronary graft conduits
         b. If previous valve repair/replacement
            1. Previous incision site
               a. Lateral chest
               b. Median sternotomy
            2. Valve/annuloplasty position
               a. Aortic
               b. Mitral
               c. Tricuspid
II. Special Equipment Needs
   A. External defibrillating electrode pads
      1. These electrode pads are applied to the back, behind the right scapula, and then laterally, below the left nipple.
   B. Oscillating saw
   C. Child chest retractor
   D. Femoral cannulation tray available
   E. Femoral perfusion cannulas
      1. Arterial
      2. Venous
   F. Anterior/posterior and lateral chest films
   G. Alligator clips and pulse generator
III. Hemostasis Considerations
   A. Pledgeted sutures available
   B. Felt sheets available
   C. Fresh frozen plasma and platelets are available on physician request after cessation of cardiopulmonary bypass.
   D. Thrombin/Gelfoam/Cryoglue is available.
   E. Surgicele is available.
   F. Avitiene is available.
IV. Team Education
   A. Advanced cardiac life support

      B. Prioritizing actions of care delivered dependent on the current status of the patient
      C. Alternate routes of cardiopulmonary bypass
V. Quality Indicators for Evaluation
      A. Number of repeat cardiac surgical procedures
      B. Pertinent scheduling information
      C. Availability of special instruments and supplies
      D. Patient outcome
          1. Safety
          2. Hemodynamic status
          3. Infection rate
          4. Intraoperative mortality rate
      E. Blood/blood product utilization
      F. Team response to emergency situations

Case Management

chapter 5

Cardiac Surgery: Policy: Designated Cardiac Surgical Suite

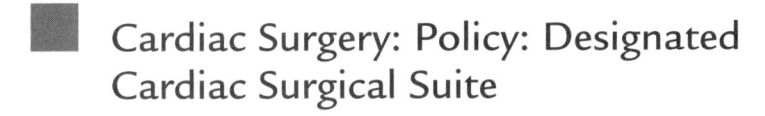

Cardiac surgery's policy is that a designated surgical suite be reserved at all times with the required cardiovascular equipment and supplies for elective and emergent cardiothoracic surgery.

Cardiac Surgical Suite

Cardiac surgical suites are designated operating rooms used exclusively for cardiac surgical procedures and invasive cardiac cath lab procedures requiring cardiac surgical team standby. These designated cardiac surgical suites must be available at all times for elective and emergent cardiac surgical procedures. The surgical table is prepared with noninvasive monitoring equipment organized for quick application. Certain characteristics are common to cardiac surgical suites. An open-heart room is built to accommodate the surgical team and special equipment. Usually six to seven people are in the room during each case. The room temperature is maintained at approximately 68°F.

This specialized suite is equipped with the current monitors and machines necessary to perform cardiac surgical procedures safely and efficiently. The equipment in this suite must be available at all times and does not move from room to room. All equipment is checked before a surgical procedure to ensure that it is available, functional, and safe. All flat surfaces are damp dusted every morning. Equipment includes but is not limited to

A. Two electrocautery units
B. A defibrillator, connected to electrical power and fully charged
C. A heart–lung machine
D. An anesthesia machine/clean anesthesia circuits
E. A slush machine
F. A K-thermia machine
G. An autotransfusion machine (cell saver)
H. Infusion pumps
I. Sitting stools
J. High and low lifts to stand on for better visualization of the surgical field
K. A hemodynamic monitor and slave monitor
L. Headlights and light sources

Special consideration is given to the electrical system to enable the use of the extensive equipment. Emergency electrical outlets are used for the most critical equipment so that intraoperative care is not compromised if the electrical power fails. Equipment is positioned in the room for quick and safe accessibility during an open-heart case. Electrical cords are kept off the floor for safety, to facilitate case flow, and to prevent damage to the cords by compression and contamination.

Good lighting is essential in a cardiac surgical suite. Usually there are three overhead table lights that are checked before surgery to ensure that all bulbs are working. Replacement bulbs are located in the surgical suite for easy and quick replacement if it becomes necessary. Overhead lights are damp dusted daily. Any malfunction with the lights or abnormalities related to the ability to focus or move the lights is reported immediately.

Headlights with their corresponding light sources are available for the surgeon's use.

Emergency lighting is available in the surgical suite and checked on a routine basis. Flashlights are kept near the heart–lung machine, in the anesthesia machine, and in a nearby prep stand.

Supplies are located in the surgical suite where delivery and use is maximized. Supplies kept in the surgical suite reflect type of cases, volume of cases, physicians' practice, and changes in technology. It is the responsibility of all team members to keep the surgical suite stocked with the pertinent items. A case cart with the supplies needed for a cardiac surgical procedure is left in the suite at all times, ready for the next elective or emergent case. Cardiosupportive drugs and IV supplies are available in the cardiac surgical suite for immediate use. The usual doses and method of delivery are posted for quick reference. Narcotics are retrieved before the surgical procedure per the request of the anesthesiologist. Volume expanders and crystalloid solutions are also stored in the cardiac surgical suite.

Good communication throughout the cardiac team is essential for quality patient care. Physician preference cards are nearby for quick reference. A current locator file is kept in the cardiac surgical suite to facilitate the location of a specific item. Cardiac surgical case documentation sheets and pertinent lab sheets are kept in the surgical suite for quick accessibility. A communication book is located on a supply cart or prep stand and is a source of information for new or broken equipment, surgeon requests, or current cardiac surgery information. An updated phone list of those units or physicians called most frequently is placed near the phone. A cardiac surgery procedure book is also kept in the room. Each type of open-heart procedure is logged along with the name of the patient and team members involved, date, implant information, and complications.

Effective organization of the surgical suite can have a substantial impact on a patient's outcome where time is of the essence. Coordinated teamwork is necessary to ensure that the cardiac surgical suite is ready at all times to meet these demands.

■ Cardiac Surgery: Policy: Organization of Supplies and Equipment in the Cardiac Surgical Suite

Cardiac surgery's policy is that the cardiac surgical suite be organized with consideration of the following criteria:

1. Backup surgical supplies are stocked in the surgical suite or in very close proximity to the surgical suite.
2. Supplies are organized for quick and easy accessibility to facilitate surgical intervention.
3. There are designated clean and contaminated areas for supplies and trash.
4. Equipment is organized to facilitate its specific use, intraoperatively, and for patient and personnel safety.
5. Traffic patterns are established to diminish the risk of contamination from outside of the surgical suite to the inside of the surgical suite.
6. Infection control measures
7. Flexibility depending on the specific surgical procedure and the needs of the patient and surgeon

Efficiency is optimized by creating realistic traffic and work-flow patterns for the patient, personnel, supplies, and equipment.

Cardiac Surgery: Nursing Procedure: Cardiac Surgical Suite Organization

Quality Outcome: The surgical suite is organized with equipment and supplies to optimize efficiency by creating realistic traffic and work-flow patterns for the personnel to facilitate patient care delivery.

Performed by: Circulating nurses, scrub nurse, hemodynamic monitoring technician, and perfusionist

General Statement: The room organization of supplies and equipment takes into consideration the components of infection control, patient and personnel safety, and efficient use of personnel, time, and effort.

Equipment: Standard cardiac surgical equipment and standard cardiac surgical supplies

Steps:	Rationale:
1. All supplies needed during a cardiac surgical procedure are stored in the surgical suite or in near proximity.	Time is life when dealing with cardiac surgical patients. Having the supplies in the surgical suite saves time and helps eliminate traffic in and out of the surgical suite.
2. Work and storage areas are provided for all types of supplies and equipment. Clean and sterile items are separated from soiled items and trash.	Separation of clean from contaminated items facilitates good aseptic technique.
3. Supplies and equipment are placed in close proximity to the location that they are needed most frequently.	Efficiency is diminished if the correlation between the space and function or time and space is great. Equipment or cables from the sterile field must be able to reach the corresponding equipment without causing a safety hazard.
4. The room is organized for optimal patient and staff safety with efficient use of personnel, time, and effort.	The goal is to make the team self-sufficient, excluding the contamination from the outside traffic to the inside of the surgical suite.

Standard of Care: Cardiac Surgery: Cardiac Surgical Suite Organization

I. Organization for Maximum Patient Safety
   A. Infection control
      1. Established traffic patterns from outside to inside the surgical suite
      2. Separation of clean from contaminated areas of the surgical suite
   B. Ease and efficiency in the transfer of the patient to and from the surgical suite
      1. Equipment is positioned around the periphery of the room.
      2. Electrical cords are affixed so that they do not run across the floors, inhibiting the patient transfer or equipment positioning, or cause a safety hazard.
II. Organization of Supplies and Equipment to Facilitate Maximum Team Efficiency
   A. Supplies
      1. Cardiac case supplies are located in the surgical suite and in close proximity to where they are used.
         a. Perfusion supplies are located in near proximity to the heart–lung machine and the sterile field.
         b. Anesthesia supplies are organized in an anesthesia supply cart at the head of the table.
         c. Cardiovascular drugs are located in the anesthesia cart and/or in a cupboard near the head of the table.
         d. Sutures are located near the surgical back table for quick retrieval.
   B. Equipment
      1. Location in the surgical suite is dependent on
         a. Type of equipment
         b. How and where it is used
         c. Time and duration of use
         d. Versatility of location to meet the needs of the patient, surgeon, and specific procedure performed
      2. Safety
         a. Equipment is positioned in close proximity to electrical outlets to decrease the risk of stumbling or inadvertent disconnection of the equipment.
III. Clinical Indicators for Evaluation
   A. Patients can be transferred in and out of the surgical suite safely and efficiently
   B. Availability of necessary supplies
   C. Accessibility of necessary supplies

- D. Positioning of the equipment meets the intraoperative needs of the patient, surgeon, and procedure performed
- E. Established traffic flow patterns to facilitate effective surgical intervention
- F. Infection control
  - a. Conduit harvesting instruments are placed at the foot of the bed or separated to one side of the instrument back table.
  - b. The mayo stand organized with the median sternotomy instruments is placed over the middle of the table.
- G. After completion of the conduit harvesting procedure, the mayo stand with the vein harvesting/radial artery harvesting instruments is moved to the periphery of the room.
  1. A sterile drape is placed over the lower legs.
  2. The vein/radial artery harvesting instruments are kept sterile until the end of the procedure.

IV. Postoperative Procedure
- A. Dressings are applied.
- B. Drapes are removed.
- C. Instrumentation and the back table of supplies are positioned at the periphery of the room and kept sterile until the patient has been transferred to the intensive care unit.
- D. The instruments are separated into basins to prevent damage.
- E. Water and disinfectant are added to the basins of instruments.
- F. The instruments are transported to the decontamination area.

V. Quality Indicators for Evaluation
- A. Availability of needed supplies and instrumentation
- B. Infection rate
- C. Case flow and turnover time
- D. Surgical time

Standard of Care: Standard Cardiac Surgical Equipment

I. Storage of Standard Cardiac Equipment
   A. Equipment remains in the cardiac surgical suite at all times for elective and emergent cardiac surgical procedures.
II. Monitoring Equipment
   A. EKG and pressure monitor with wave-form display with the capability of lead changes
   B. Noninvasive blood pressure monitor
   C. Pulse oximeter monitor and probe
   D. CO_2 monitor
   E. SVO_2 monitor
   F. Cardiac output monitor
   G. Transport monitor
   H. Temperature monitor
III. Autotransfusion Equipment
   A. Cell saver processor
   B. Autotransfusion system
   C. Blood warmer
   D. Heart–lung machine
   E. Blood refrigerator or ice chest for bank blood storage
   F. Hemoconcentration system
IV. Electrical Conduction Equipment
   A. DC defibrillator and internal paddles
   B. External defibrillating pads with the corresponding cable adaptor to connect to the defibrillator
   C. Electrical fibrillator and corresponding electrodes
   D. External and internal pulse pacemaker generator, single and dual chamber
   E. Epicardial pacemaker leads, temporary and permanent
   F. Internal, implantable defibrillator with the corresponding leads
V. Mechanical Assist Devices
   A. Mechanical assist pumps
   B. Intra-aortic balloon pump
   C. Intra-aortic balloons
VI. Stat Lab Equipment
   A. ACT I HPT machine
   B. Blood gas analysis machine
   C. Blood glucose machine
   D. Electrolyte analysis machine

VII. Miscellaneous Equipment
    A. Fiberoptic headlight and light source
    B. Thermia unit
    C. Two electrocautery units
    D. Standing stools
    E. Slush machine

VIII. Clinical Indicators for Evaluation
    A. Availability of equipment
    B. Staff education
        1. Equipment required
        2. Functioning and use
        3. Proper maintenance

Cardiac Surgery: Policy: Preparation of the Sterile Field

Cardiac surgery's policy is that the implementation of a sterile field in preparation for organizing the sterile instruments and supplies needed for the cardiac surgical procedure meets the following criteria:

1. Sterile supplies and instrumentation are opened and organized no earlier than an hour before the scheduled surgical time.
2. The sterile field is never left unattended.
3. The integrity of the sterile field is maintained until the patient is safely transferred to the intensive care unit.

Cardiac Surgery: Nursing Procedure: Preparation of the Sterile Field

Quality Outcome: A sterile field is created to facilitate the preparation and maintain the aseptic integrity of the instruments and supplies needed during a cardiac surgical procedure.

Performed by: Surgical scrub nurse

General Statement: The supplies and instruments are not opened and organized any earlier than an hour before the scheduled surgical time.

The supplies and instrumentation are checked against the physician's preference card for the specific procedure.

Equipment: Instrument table, one to two mayo stands, two single-ring stands, one double-ring stand, appropriate instrument trays for the scheduled procedure, custom packs, suture material, and perfusion table circuits

Steps:	Rationale:
1. The scrub nurse checks the case cart for appropriate supplies and equipment using the physician's preference card as a reference. The integrity of the packaging is inspected.	Supplies needed for the procedure are available and sterile.
2. The basic custom pack is opened on the back table. Additional custom packs are opened on ring stands.	The covered back table creates a sterile field on which to work.
3. Heavy instrument trays are opened on the ring stands.	The ring stands can support the weight of the instrument trays.
4. All small packages are opened in basins or instrument trays, leaving the back table free of excess supplies.	Facilitates setup time when supplies do not have to be moved several times.
5. The perfusion table pump circuit is opened and placed in an instrument tray or basin.	The perfusion circuit is opened on the field in a location where it will not fall, becoming contaminated.

Steps:	Rationale:
6. The scrub nurse dons sterile gown and gloves to organize the sterile supplies and instruments.	The scrub nurse's responsibility is for the preparation of the sterile field.
7. The back table is covered with an extra drape sheet, paper, or linen.	The extra drape provides protection to prevent tears in the back table cover from instrument trays with resulting contamination.
8. The instrument trays are placed on the back table. The scrub nurse and circulating nurse complete the required sponge, needle, and instrument counts.	Initial counts provide a baseline for subsequent counts.
9. The mayo stand(s) is draped. Instruments needed for the median sternotomy and cardiopulmonary bypass are placed on a mayo stand. If a CABG procedure is to be performed, the vein-harvesting instruments are organized on a second mayo stand.	The instrumentation for the median sternotomy is separate from the instruments used for conduit harvesting to prevent wound cross-contamination.
10. The supplies are organized on the back table. All paper and caps are removed from the supplies and disposed of properly.	Unintended retention of a foreign substance in the body may cause physical damage to the patient.
11. The surgical drapes are organized in the order that they are to be used.	Facilitates the draping procedure.
12. The integrity of the sterile field is maintained until the patient has been transferred to the intensive care unit.	If the patient becomes hemodynamically unstable during the transfer, the mediastinum may be re-explored.

Standard of Care: Cardiac Surgery: Sterile Field Preparation

I. Preoperative Case Preparation
   A. Case organization
      1. The physician preference card is used to verify the correct supplies and instrumentation.
         a. The scrub nurse checks the case cart for the correct supplies and instrumentation.
   B. The scrub nurse/tech and circulating nurses complete the preliminary housekeeping in the surgical suite.
   C. The scrub nurse/tech opens the sterile supplies and instruments 1 hour before the surgical procedure.
      1. The basic custom pack is opened on the back table.
      2. The instruments are placed on ring stands.
      3. Extra supplies are opened in basins or instrument trays.
      4. Sutures are opened in basins or instrument trays.
   D. The scrub nurse/tech scrubs his/her hands and dons a gown and gloves.
      1. An extra drape sheet is placed over the back table for protection.
      2. The instruments are placed on the back table.
      3. The supplies are organized on the back table.
      4. The initial sponge, needle, and instrument counts are completed.
      5. The mayo stand/stands are draped.
         a. The instrumentation and suture needed for the median sternotomy and cardiopulmonary bypass are organized on the first mayo stand.
         b. The instruments needed for the vein-harvesting procedure are organized on a second mayo stand or to the side of the instrument table for easy access.
      6. All drapes are organized in order of use.
II. Intraoperative Preparations
   A. The patient is draped according to the procedure for the specific type of case.
   B. The sterile lines and equipment are passed from the surgical field to their appropriate terminals.
      1. Electrocautery for the median sternotomy
      2. The autotransfusion aspiration circuit
      3. Internal paddles
      4. Sternal saw
      5. Electrocautery for the vein-harvesting procedure

6. Perfusion table circuits
   a. The circuits are passed from the sterile field to the perfusionist, who then connects the circuits to the heart–lung machine.
7. The mayo stands are moved up to the surgical table.
   a. The mayo stand organized with the vein-harvesting instruments is placed at the foot of the bed.
   b. The mayo stand organized with the median sternotomy instruments is placed over the middle of the table.
   C. After completion of the conduit-harvesting procedure, the mayo stand is moved to the periphery of the room.
   1. A sterile drape is placed over the lower legs.
   2. The conduit-harvesting instruments are kept sterile until the end of the procedure.
III. Postoperative Procedure
   A. Dressings are applied.
   B. Drapes are removed.
   C. Instrumentation and the back table of supplies are positioned at the periphery of the room and kept sterile until the patient has been transferred to the intensive care unit.
   D. The instruments are separated into basins to prevent damage.
   E. Water and disinfectant are added to the basins of instruments.
   F. The instruments are transported to the decontamination area.
IV. Quality Indicators for Evaluation
   A. Availability of needed supplies and instrumentation
   B. Infection rate
   C. Case flow and turnover time
   D. Surgical time
   E. Scheduling conflicts

Cardiac Surgery: Policy: Instrument Inventory Management

Cardiac surgery's policy is that an instrument count sheet be placed in every instrument tray for the following purposes:

1. Aid to assure proper instrumentation per tray
2. Assist with organization of the instruments in the tray
3. Document any discrepancies of amounts and types of instrumentation perioperatively
4. Doubles as the count sheet for the operative procedure

Cardiac Surgery: Nursing Procedure: Instrument Inventory Management

Quality Outcome: The surgical team will initiate an instrument monitoring system to facilitate patient safety that will assure the availability of needed instruments, ensure their optimum functioning capability, and prevent their loss.

Performed by: Scrub nurse, circulating nurse, and instrument room personnel

General Statement: Each instrument tray is monitored for correct instrumentation per tray along with inspection of the integrity of the individual instruments before the surgical procedure begins.

Equipment: Instrument trays, instrument count sheets

Steps:	Rationale:
1. Instrument trays are organized to meet physician's preference, type of procedure, size of patient, and AORN standards.	Correct instrumentation is assured. Guidelines for effective sterilization requirements are met.
2. Instruments are inspected for damage and are counted and documented on the individual trays' count sheets in the instrument reprocessing unit.	Baseline instrumentation inventory is obtained.
3. Damaged instruments are replaced.	Instruments are functional and intact.
4. Instruments are arranged in a specific pattern.	Reducing the amount and types of instruments and streamlining sets facilitates the counting process. Instruments are organized to prevent damage.
5. The instrument count sheet is placed inside the tray prior to sterilization. Missing instruments are documented on the count sheet.	Any discrepancies are noted, alerting the surgical team before the surgical procedure.
6. The name of the staff member organizing the instrument tray and date is documented on the instrument count sheet.	Facilitates further investigation if necessary.

Steps:	Rationale:
7. The scrub nurse submits the instrument count sheet to the circulating nurse. All instruments are exposed and inspected for their integrity and functional capability. Detachable or disassembled parts are added to the count.	Scrub and circulating nurse complete the instrument count, preoperatively. All instrument parts must be accounted for.
8. Any instrumentation added to the sterile field during the procedure is added to the count sheet. Instruments that fall from the sterile field are replaced or, if not needed, retained to be able to combine them with the sterile field count. Pieces of broken instruments are recovered and retained. Replacement instruments are added to the count.	The instrument count is kept up to date, throughout the procedure. All instruments are accounted for in their entirety.
9. Subsequent counts are taken when scrub nurses are relieved during a case and before closure of the mediastinum.	It is the responsibility of the circulator and scrub nurse to complete the required instrument counts.
10. Instrument counts are documented on the operative record as correct or incorrect by the circulating nurse and reported to the surgeon.	Final outcome of counts is documented in writing.
11. Incorrect counts necessitate another count, with a thorough search of trash, floor, and OR suite, field, and wound. An x-ray is taken before the patient leaves the OR suite if the instrument is still missing. An incident report is completed.	All attempts are made to locate the missing instrument. Actions are documented to verify that all attempts were made to find the missing item.
12. The final instrument count sheet is sent along with the instruments to the instrument reprocessing unit.	Will alert the instrument processing staff of any missing or broken instruments.

Standard of Care: Cardiac Surgery: Instrument Inventory Management

I. Instrument Tray Organization
   A. Meets the needs of the surgeon and procedure
   B. Meets sterilization requirements
      1. Steam
         a. Steam penetration
         b. Revaporization for drying
         c. Meets weight requirements
      2. Gas
         a. Aeration requirements if ETOH
         b. Hydrogen peroxide gas
   C. Protection from damage
   D. Ease in removal, setup, counting, and use
II. Perioperative Instrument Counts
   A. Instruments counted and organized by instrument processing personnel
      1. Instrument inventory sheet placed in each instrument tray
      2. Discrepancies noted or missing instruments replaced
   B. Scrub and circulating nurses complete the instrument count before surgical procedure
      1. Discrepancies noted
      2. Instruments' condition and functioning ability checked
      3. Missing instruments documented
      4. Malfunctioning instruments are replaced and sent for repair
   C. Scrub and circulating nurse complete instrument count after cessation of extracorporeal circulation and reapproximation of the sternum
      1. Instrument count documented on the surgical record as correct or incorrect
   D. Missing instruments are accounted for in their entirety.
      1. The circulating nurse notifies the scrub nurse of instruments off of the sterile field.
      2. The surgical suite is searched if there is a missing instrument.
      3. X-rays are taken before patient transport, if the nurses are unable to locate the missing instrument.
   E. Instrument count sheets are returned with the dirty instruments to the instrument processing area.
      1. Discrepancies noted
      2. Instruments needing repair are marked accordingly, stating the type of repair needed.

III. Special Instrument Inventory
   A. Manufacturer
   B. Catalog number
   C. Cost
   D. Maintenance
   E. Warranty
   F. Sterilization procedure
   G. Staff education
      1. Care and handling
      2. Use
      3. Locator file or electronic instrument management system for instrument tray location
IV. Basic Cardiac Instrument Trays
   A. Basic cardiac tray
   B. Vein/radial harvesting/CABG tray
   C. Valve tray
   D. Thoracic tray
   E. Femoral cannulation tray
   F. Sternal rewiring tray
   G. Intensive care emergency chest set
V. Quality Indicators for Evaluation
   A. Instrumentation handling, storage, and processing meets AORN guidelines
   B. Availability of instrumentation
   C. Efficacy of instrumentation tray organization; meeting the need to which it is intended
   D. Time management of instrument case organization, counting, and reprocessing

■ Cardiac Surgery: Policy: Cardiac Supply Inventory

Cardiac surgery's policy is that all cardiac supplies be managed by the cardiac manager to maintain adequate inventory of the necessary items. A supply log is maintained containing information including, but not limited to, the following:

1. Name of the manufacturer
2. Catalog numbers
3. How the product is supplied
4. Cost of the supplies
5. Date supplies ordered
6. Date order received
7. Lot numbers

All requisitions for supplies must be signed by the cardiac manager.

Cardiac Surgery Nursing Procedure: Requisition of Cardiac Surgical Supplies

Quality Outcome: Adequate inventory of cardiac surgical supplies is maintained and documented.

Performed by: Cardiac team member/cardiac surgery manager

General Statement: All requisitions for supplies are signed by the cardiac surgery manager. A supply log is maintained.

Equipment: Supply log

Steps:

1. The cardiac surgery manager completes the appropriate requisition form to place an order for supplies. Information includes, but is not limited to, the following:
   a. Manufacturer
   b. Catalog or model number
   c. Amount needed
   d. Date of order
   e. Department where the order originated

2. The supply log documentation includes, but is not limited to, the following:
   a. Manufacturer
   b. Catalog or model number
   c. Amount of item ordered
   d. Date of order
   e. Cost of item

Rationale:

Inventory is controlled and the appropriate supplies are available for a cardiac surgical case.

The supply log provides information needed for utilization review and future reference should a question arise regarding the ordered item.

Steps:	Rationale:

3. When the items have been received from the purchasing department, they are compared with the ordering requisition. Charge stickers are applied, if applicable. The following is documented in the supply log:
   a. Date order arrived
   b. Complete or incomplete order
   c. Lot numbers of the ordered items
	The order received is checked against the order requisitioned to ensure that the order is complete. Lot numbers are documented in case there are any problems or complications arising from the use of the items.

4. Current records are maintained.	Facilitates the ordering process.
5. The inventory of supplies is rotated and checked for sterility.	Stocked supplies are rotated to decrease the incidence of outdates.
6. Supply recall notification from manufacturers is checked against the current inventory. The recalled products are sent back to the manufacturer according to their instructions.	Documentation of the lot numbers aids in tracking the items recalled. Recalled items are unsafe for use and must be returned to the manufacturer as soon as notified.

Standard of Care: Cardiac Surgery: Supply Management

I. Inventory Record of Supplies
   A. Manufacturer name
   B. Item number, model number, lot numbers
   C. How item is supplied, cost, and amount ordered
   D. Time needed to receive order
   E. Date order sent
   F. Date order received; order complete or incomplete
   G. Product evaluation
II. Inventory of Special Equipment
   A. Manufacturer
   B. Operation manual
   C. Model and serial numbers
   D. Cost of equipment, maintenance records, and warranties
   E. Locator file for location of specific supplies
III. Standardization of Supplies
   A. Custom packs
      1. Major CV pack
      2. Vein/radial harvesting pack
      3. Suture packs
      4. Perfusion packs
   B. Anesthesia invasive line supplies/fluids/drugs
   C. Valve inventory
      1. Mechanical
      2. Biological
      3. Annuloplasty rings
      4. Valve graft conduits
   D. Special cardiac implants
      1. Intraluminal synthetic vascular grafts
      2. Intra-aortic balloons
      3. Internal defibrillators
      4. Ventricular assist devices
      5. Gott shunts
      6. Permanent pacemakers
IV. Case Cost Documentation
   A. Case charges itemized
      1. All chargeable items appropriately labeled
      2. Standard case charge system
   B. Product research and cost evaluation

          1. Function
          2. Use
          3. Safety
          4. Quality
          5. Cost
    C. Standardization of supplies
V. Clinical Indicators for Evaluation
    A. Appropriate documentation and record keeping
    B. Supply cost
    C. Supply utilization
    D. Availability of supplies

Preoperative Preparation

chapter 6

■ Cardiac Surgery: Policy: Perioperative Nursing Assessment of the Cardiac Surgical Patient

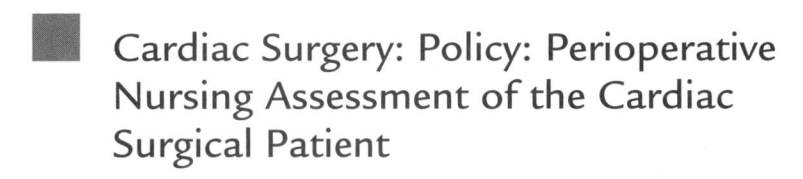

Cardiac surgery's policy is that a perioperative nursing assessment be completed to facilitate the intraoperative plan of care for the cardiac surgical patient, increasing the probability of desired patient outcomes.

The assessment includes but is not limited to the following:

1. Physiological status
2. Psychosocial status

The plan of care is continually redesigned to meet the changing needs of the cardiac surgical patient.

Physical Assessment of the Cardiac Surgical Patient

The physical assessment of the cardiac surgical patient provides the perioperative nurse with the baseline data and pertinent history to analyze potential problems and plan appropriate interventions should they be required. It is essential that the perioperative nurse communicate this assessment data to the healthcare team to assure continuity of care.

Inspection, auscultation, and palpation are integrated into the five areas of assessment, which include

A. Integumentary status
B. Level of mentation
C. Nutritional status
D. Respiratory status
E. Circulatory status

I. Integumentary Status
   Assessment of the integumentary status of the cardiac patient can reflect impaired vascular function and also the potential for infection for the postoperative cardiac surgical patient.
   A. Evaluation of the color of the skin
      1. Pallor
      2. Flushing
      3. Cyanosis
      4. Petechiae
      5. Jaundice
   B. Temperature of skin
      1. Presence of coolness
      2. Presence of clamminess
      3. Diaphoresis
   C. Evaluation of the extremities
      1. Capillary filling
      2. Absence of extremities or digits
      3. Motor impairments
      4. Neck vein distension
      5. Edema
         a. Quality
         b. Extent
      6. Sensory impairments
      7. Clubbing of the fingers

   8. Varicose veins
   9. Peripheral pulses
  D. Evaluation of the integrity of the skin
   1. Open sores or lesions
   2. Type of scars and locations

II. Nutritional Status

The baseline nutritional assessment of the cardiac surgical patient can give valuable information needed to handle this type of patient proactively both preoperatively and postoperatively.

  A. Weight
   1. Obesity
   2. Malnourished
   3. Anorexic
  B. Diet
   1. Culture
    a. Body image
   2. Culinary habits
    a. Herbal concoctions
    b. Vitamin use
   3. Level of education
  C. Underlying physical conditions
   1. Diabetes
  D. Levels of activity
   1. Exercises regularly
   2. Sedentary
   3. Exercise intolerant

III. Levels of Mentation

The levels of mentation of a patient not only play a vital role in how well a patient comprehends his or her course of treatment but also lend valuable clues to underlying emotional or physical complications.

  A. Level of consciousness
   1. Responsive
   2. Unresponsive
  B. Patient's ability to respond appropriately
   1. Language barrier
   2. Level of comprehension
    a. Patient's level of knowledge regarding surgical intervention
    b. Patient's cultural and religious beliefs
   3. Sensory impairment
   4. Level of expression
  C. Emotional status
   1. Anxiety

        2. Depressed
            a. Coping mechanisms
    D. Pain
        1. Location
        2. Occurrence
        3. Tolerance
        4. Type and intensity
        5. Effective pain-relief measures
    E. Respiratory status
        1. Hypoxic
    F. Dental care
IV. Respiratory Status
The respiratory system has a direct influence over the quality of function for the entire body by controlling ventilation and perfusion of oxygen.
    A. Patient's history
        1. Work patterns
            a. Exposure to pollutants
            b. Levels of activity
        2. Occurrence and frequency of infectious or inflammatory disease
        3. History of smoking
        4. COPD
        5. Previous thoracic surgery
            a. Lobectomy, thoracoscopy
                1. History of radiation
    B. Physical mechanics of breathing
        1. Observation of chest wall movement
            a. Inspiration/expiration
                1. Ease/difficulty
                    a. Use of accessory breathing muscles in the chest or neck
                    b. Special positional requirements
                    c. Presence of pain
        2. Ratio between inspiration/expiration
        3. Symmetry of chest
    C. Auscultation of breath sounds
        1. Location
            a. Presence or absence
            b. Comparison from one side of the chest to another
        2. Quality
            a. Clear/muffled
                1. Wheezing
                2. Rhonchi/rales
                3. Pleural friction rub

4. Presence of a cough
       b. Nonproductive
       c. Productive
             1. Amount
             2. Color
             3. Consistency
    D. Rate/rhythm and depth of respirations
    E. Physical appearance
       1. Color
       2. Level of mentation
    F. Lab values
       1. Chest x-ray
       2. Pulmonary function tests
       3. ABGS
       4. CBC
V. Circulatory System
   This system is responsible for transportation of oxygen and nutrients to the cells of the body.
    A. Patient's history
       1. General appearance
          a. Color of skin
          b. Temperature of skin
          c. Perfusion
          d. Sensation
       2. Nutritional status
          a. Fluid volume
       3. Mentation
       4. Activity
       5. Underlying physical conditions
          a. Hypertension, hyperlipidemia
          b. PVD
          c. Previous cardiac surgery
          d. Pacemaker, internal defibrillator
       6. Current medications
    B. Cardiac function
       1. Cardiac cath lab report
          a. Evaluation of heart function
             1. Ejection fraction
             2. Cardiac output
             3. Coronary circulation
          b. Visualization of heart chambers
             1. Ventricle hypertrophy

Physical Assessment of the Cardiac Surgical Patient

    2. Aneurysms
   c. Measurements of intracardiac pressures
    1. Valve competency
    2. Shunts
   d. Hemodynamic parameters
    1. Peripheral BP
    2. PA pressures
    3. CVP
    4. SVR
 C. Palpation of pulses
  1. Location
  2. Presence/absence
   a. Quality
    1. Weak
    2. Bounding
    3. Equality of pulses
   b. Rate
    1. Fast
    2. Slow
    3. Patient's response to the rate
  3. Rhythm
   a. Regular
   b. Irregular
    1. Patient's response to dysrhythmias
 D. Auscultation of heartbeat
  1. Quality
   a. Clear
   b. Muffled
   c. Presence of murmurs
  2. Location of heart sounds
 E. Lab values
  1. CBC
  2. Electrolytes
  3. Cardiac enzymes
  4. BUN
  5. PT/PTT
  6. EKG

Cardiac Surgery: Nursing Procedure: Perioperative Nursing Assessment of the Cardiac Surgical Patient

Quality Outcome: The nursing assessment provides the cardiac team with baseline information about potential problems that might require intervention.
Performed by: Circulating nurses, scrub nurse, perfusionist, and hemodynamic monitoring specialist
General Statement: Assessment of the patient should be comprehensive because cardiac function affects all of the body's systems.
Equipment: Patient chart

Steps:	Rationale:
1. The circulating nurse identifies the patient and introduces himself or herself before transfer of the patient to the surgical suite.	The patient's identity is confirmed.
2. The circulating nurse initiates the nursing assessment by reading the documentation of the patient's history and lab results found in the chart.	The lab results are screened for any abnormalities or deletions.
3. The circulating nurse assesses the patient's physiological and psychosocial status using the following techniques: a. Inspection/observation b. Palpation c. Percussion d. Olfaction e. Subjective	The nursing assessment provides the team with baseline data and information regarding potential problems that might require intervention.

Steps:	Rationale:

4. All of the major body systems are assessed, including but not limited to
   a. Integumentary
   b. Circulatory
   c. Respiratory
   d. Neurological
   e. Musculoskeletal
	Cardiac function affects all of the body's organ systems. A comprehensive assessment of the patient alerts the team to any potential problems.

5. Attainable goals are established to meet the specific needs of the patient using the standards of care as guidelines.	Specific actions are established using the standards of care as guidelines. Standards of care describe the kind of care patients can expect to receive from the nursing staff.
6. The action plans are implemented, prioritizing actions to meet the goals. The patient's response to the action taken is monitored and evaluated.	Goals are revised, as needed, to meet the specific needs of the patient.
7. Documentation of the nursing assessment, actions taken to meet the required goals, and the patient's response to those actions implemented are documented on the surgical record.	Documentation accurately reflects assessment, planning, perioperative care given, and evaluation of outcomes.

Standard of Care: Cardiac Surgery: Perioperative Nursing Assessment of the Cardiac Surgical Patient

I. Perioperative Nursing Function
   A. Assessment
      1. Physiological
      2. Psychosocial
   B. Planning
      1. Establishment of attainable goals to meet the specific needs of the patient
   C. Implementation
      1. Assessment and determination of priorities
      2. Continuous reassessment
      3. Goal modifications to meet the changing needs of the patient
   D. Evaluation
      1. Clinical indicators to facilitate the evaluation process

II. Physiologic Assessment
   A. Techniques
      1. Inspection/observation
         a. Skin
            1. Color and integrity
            2. Allergies
            3. Nutritional and metabolic status
            4. Height and weight
            5. Mobility
            6. Altercations from previous surgery, injury, or disease
            7. Presence of edema
            8. Diaphoresis
         b. Prosthetics
            1. Internal
            2. External
         c. Medical diagnosis
            1. Operative site and procedure
            2. Results of laboratory tests and diagnostic studies
            3. Vital signs
            4. Current medications
            5. NPO status
         d. Respiratory assessment
            1. Neck vein distension

            2. Shortness of breath
        2. Palpation
            a. Presence of pulses
                1. Rate
                2. Rhythm
                3. Quality
            b. Blood pressure
                1. High, low, or normal pressure
                2. Equal blood pressures bilaterally
        3. Percussion
            a. Auscultation of breath sounds
                1. Unilateral or bilateral
                    a. Intensity
                    b. Quality
                    c. Rate
            b. Auscultation of heart sounds
                1. Quality
                2. Rate
                3. Rhythm
                4. Olfaction
                5. Subjective
                    a. Sensory impairments
                    b. Presence of pain
                        1. Type
                        2. Location
                        3. Duration
                        4. Intensity
                        5. Mechanism that relieves pain
III. Psychosocial Considerations
    A. Emotional
        1. Expectation of care
        2. Support from family
        3. Nonverbal behavior
        4. Cultural and religious beliefs
            a. Jehovah's Witness
    B. Cognition
        1. Speech characteristics
            a. Language barrier
            b. Speech deficit
            c. Level of comprehension
        2. Stress level
            a. Presence of fear or anxiety

                1. Identifying contributing factors
          b. Coping mechanisms
                1. Attitude
                2. Motivation

IV. Planning the Perioperative Care
    A. Established standard of care
        1. Specific actions to achieve goals
        2. Set priorities for goal attainment
        3. Role responsibilities for implementation of goals
        4. When, where, and how the goals are attained

V. Implementation
    A. Standard of care is implemented.
        1. Individualized to meet the specific needs of the patient
        2. Goal directed
    B. The patient's responses are continually monitored.
        1. Goals are revised to meet the patient's needs.

VI. Clinical Indicators for Evaluation
    A. Patient responses to nursing intervention
        1. Expected results
        2. Actual results
    B. Staff accountability
        1. Continuing education
        2. Nursing research
    C. Documentation
        1. Results of planned nursing action
        2. Revisions of plans based on the reassessment of the patient's needs

Cardiac Surgery: Policy: Preoperative Lab Procedures

Cardiac surgery's policy is that the physician order the preoperative lab procedures for the cardiac surgical patient. The completed lab results are recorded on the chart and screened for omissions or abnormalities by the circulating nurse before transport of the patient to the surgical suite. Abnormalities or omissions are brought to the attention of the physician.

Cardiac Surgery: Nursing Procedure: Assessment of the Preoperative Lab Procedures

Quality Outcome: The cardiac surgical procedure is preceded by extensive cardiovascular assessments using noninvasive and invasive studies that dictate subsequent care.
Performed by: Surgeon, lab personnel, and circulating nurse
General Statement: The circulating nurse assesses the preoperative orders for the completion of the necessary preoperative tests and screens the results for any abnormalities before transporting the patient to the surgical suite.
Equipment: Not applicable

Steps:

1. The circulating nurse introduces himself or herself to the patient.

2. The circulating nurse assesses the chart for completeness using the physician's preoperative orders as a reference. The following tests have been completed and the results are documented, including but not limited to
   a. CBC
   b. Urinalysis
   c. Electrolytes
   d. Chest x-ray
   e. EKG
   f. Blood type and cross-match
   g. Coag panel
   h. Pulmonary function tests, if warranted
   i. BUN and creatinine

Rationale:

The nurse verifies the correct identification of the patient and tries to establish a sense of trust with the patient to alleviate some of the preoperative anxiety.

An extensive cardiovascular assessment is used to facilitate subsequent treatment. All lab determinations are on the chart before the operative procedure to prevent unnecessary delays.

Steps:	Rationale:
3. The circulating nurse checks to ensure that the medical history and the physical and the heart catheterization report are on the chart.	The history of the patient enables the team to coordinate the intraoperative plan of care.
4. Any omissions or abnormalities of the preoperative testing are brought to the attention of the surgeon.	The surgeon's plan of care may change according to the results of the various preoperative tests.
5. The circulating nurse signs the preoperative checklist, documenting the fact that the preoperative lab preparations have been completed as ordered and that there are no discrepancies noted.	All perioperative care must be documented to meet the policies of the individual institution and JCAHO.

Standard of Care: Cardiac Surgery: Preoperative Procedures

I. Types of Preoperative Procedures
   A. Diagnostic testing
   B. Lab determinations
   C. Medical history and physical exam
II. Indications for Preoperative Procedures
   A. Adequately prepare the patient for the surgical procedure
      1. Enables the healthcare team to plan the care appropriate for the individual patient
      2. Specific tests are ordered by the surgeon for the preoperative preparations.
         a. Standard orders
         b. Orders specific for the individual patient dependent on the patient's underlying physical condition
III. Diagnostic Procedures for the Cardiac Surgical Patient
   A. Cardiac catheterization
      1. Evaluation of cardiac function
      2. Evaluation of intracardiac pressures
      3. Visualization of the heart
   B. Coronary angiograms
      1. Evaluation of coronary artery disease
      2. Extent and location of the coronary obstruction
   C. Echocardiogram
      1. Valvular disease
   D. EKG
   E. Chest x-ray
IV. Lab Determinations
   A. CBC
   B. Urinalysis
   C. Electrolytes
   D. Type and cross-match for blood
      1. Type and cross-match for the blood must be within 48–72 hrs of the surgical procedure.
   E. Pulmonary function tests
      1. Oxygen saturation tests
         a. Pulse oximeter
         b. Arterial blood gas determinations
   F. Coag panel
      1. Bleeding history

V. Medical History and Physical Exam
   A. They are completed by the surgeon before the surgical procedure.
   B. The report is documented on the patient's chart.
   C. The history and physical correlate with the surgical consent.
VI. Clinical Indicators for Evaluation
   A. Surgeon's orders are completed.
   B. Lab determinations are completed.
      1. Lab determinations are charted preoperatively.
      2. Surgery is not delayed.
      3. Lab tests are not repeated unnecessarily.
   C. The medical history and physical are on the chart preoperatively.

Patient Care Activities

chapter 7

Cardiac Surgery: Policy: Transfer of the Stable Cardiac Surgical Patient to Surgery

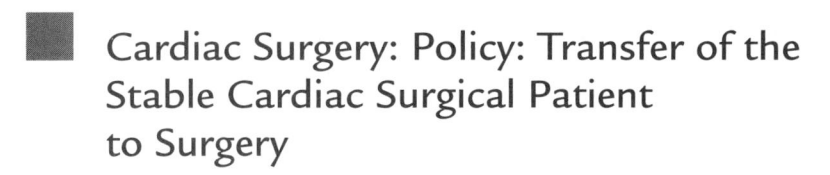

Cardiac surgery's policy is that stable, cardiac surgical patients be transported to surgery by a nursing assistant 1 hour before the scheduled surgery start time. This permits adequate time for the preoperative preparation of the cardiac patient. Cardiac monitoring and oxygen therapy during transport are instituted when ordered by the physician.

The needs for oxygen and cardiac monitoring may be reassessed when warranted by a change in the patient's physical condition.

If the patient must be continuously monitored, a licensed staff member shall accompany the transport to surgery.

Cardiac Surgery: Nursing Procedure: Transfer of the Stable Cardiac Surgical Patient to Surgery

Quality Outcome: Patients are transferred from their hospital rooms to surgery or the designated holding area safely and expediently with adequate time for preoperative preparation.

Performed by: Orderly, nursing assistant, and nursing staff

General Statement: The first patient of the day is brought directly to the surgical suite by the transporter. If surgery is delayed or if it is the second scheduled case of the day, the patient is brought to the surgical holding area.

Equipment: Gurney/bed transporter

Steps:	Rationale:
1. The circulating nurse notifies the floor or unit of the time the patient will be transferred to surgery. The circulating nurse receives a report regarding the patient's current physical condition.	Allows the unit time to prepare the patient for surgery. Facilitates the organization of the perioperative care plan.
2. The circulating nurse notifies the transporter of the patient's location, the name of the patient, and the time transfer is to occur.	Pertinent information is relayed to prevent unnecessary delays.
3. The transporter delivers the patient to the surgical suite or surgery holding area.	The first case of the day is taken directly to the surgical suite. The second case of the day is taken to the surgery holding area.
4. The circulating nurse identifies the patient, completes a preoperative nursing assessment, and checks the chart for proper documentation of lab work, consents, and diagnostic data. Any abnormalities are brought to the anesthesiologist's and surgeon's attention.	Correct patient identification is made. All lab results are documented. Each patient's need for nursing care is assessed. Any discrepancies are brought to the physician's attention.

Steps:	Rationale:
5. The patient is transferred from the gurney or bed to the surgical table. Assessment is made to determine whether the patient is capable of moving on his or her own. Patients complaining of chest pain/shortness of breath or who have a physical disability should not move themselves.	Physical exertion causes an increase in myocardial oxygen consumption. A roller can be used to transfer the patient safely.
6. Warm blankets are applied to the patient. Care is taken to relieve any patient anxiety.	Shivering causes an increase in myocardial oxygen demands. Anxiety increases myocardial oxygen consumption.
7. The surgical table safety strap is applied over the patient's thighs.	Safety strap restrains leg movement.
8. Noninvasive monitoring equipment is applied to the patient in the surgical suite and surgery holding area.	Cardiac patients are monitored continuously perioperatively.

■ Standard of Care: Cardiac Surgery: Transfer of the Stable Cardiac Patient to Surgery

I. Interdepartmental Communication
   A. Transfer of the patient
      1. The patient care unit is notified in advance of the transfer.
      2. A verbal report is given to the circulating nurse.
         a. Current physiologic status of the patient
         b. Invasive lines present
         c. Any allergies
         d. Any special concerns
      3. A preoperative checklist is completed.
      4. An orderly or nursing assistant is sent to transfer the patient to surgery.
         a. The patient is transported on a gurney.
II. Monitoring During Transport
   A. Stable patient
      1. Monitored if ordered by the surgeon
         a. If monitored, the circulating nurse accompanies the transport.
      2. Oxygen, if ordered by the surgeon
III. Transfer to the Cardiac Surgical Suite
   A. The first patient of the day is taken directly to the surgical suite.
      1. The circulating nurse properly identifies the patient, completes a nursing assessment, and reviews the chart.
      2. The preoperative checklist is checked and signed by the circulating nurse.
   B. The following cases are sent for after the first patient has been weaned from cardiopulmonary bypass and is stable.
      1. The patient is transferred from the patient care unit to the surgery holding room.
      2. After the circulating nurse has properly identified the patient and completed the preoperative assessment of the patient and chart, the patient is transferred to the cardiac surgical suite.
   C. The patient is positioned on the surgical table in preparation for invasive line placement.
   D. Noninvasive monitoring equipment is applied.
IV. Clinical Indicators for Evaluation
   A. Safety of the transfer
   B. Time needed for transfer
   C. Interdepartmental communication

Cardiac Surgery: Policy: Transfer of the Unstable Cardiac Surgical Patient to Surgery

Cardiac surgery's policy is that the following criteria be met when transporting the unstable cardiac patient.

1. The circulating nurse, hemodynamic monitoring technician, and anesthesia provider are sent to transport the patient to surgery.
2. The patient is transferred in the same bed.
3. The patient's hemodynamics are monitored: heart rate, rhythm, arterial pressure.
4. Supplemental oxygen is available, per physician's order.
5. If the patient requires mechanical ventilation, an anesthesiologist is present to assist with the transfer.
6. Extra personnel are used, as needed, for safe transportation.
7. If the intra-aortic balloon is in place, the transfer is monitored by licensed personnel certified in balloon pumping.
8. Surgical consents are complete.
9. The surgeons are available.
10. All attempts are made to expedite the surgical process.
    A. The first patient of the day is taken directly to the surgical suite.

Cardiac Surgery: Nursing Procedure: Transfer of the Unstable Cardiac Surgical Patient to Surgery

Quality Outcome: Unstable cardiac patients are transferred safely and expediently to surgery, with continuous monitoring of their hemodynamic status.
Performed by: Circulating nurse, hemodynamic monitoring specialist, and cardiac anesthesiologist
General Statement: Unstable patients are accompanied by licensed personnel during the transport to surgery with continual hemodynamic monitoring in the event that cardiac life support becomes necessary.
Equipment: Transport monitor, EKG electrodes and cables, transducer cables, and defibrillator

Steps:	Rationale:
1. The circulating nurse inquires about the cardiovascular status of the patient, the location of any invasive lines, drugs, or any mechanical assist devices.	Assists in prioritizing perioperative plan of cardiac supportive care for the cardiac surgical patient.
2. The unit is given an estimated time of patient transport to surgery.	Allows the unit time to finish documentation of care and the surgical checklist.
3. The circulatig nurse organizes extra assistance, as needed, for transfer.	Safe transfer is made.
4. The circulating nurse identifies the patient, completes a preoperative physical assessment, and checks the chart.	Proper identification is accomplished. The chart is complete, and lab results are recorded. The perioperative plan of care is reassessed when warranted by the patient's condition.

Steps:	Rationale:
5. The circulating nurse applies EKG electrodes and cables to the patient and connects them to the transport monitor. The hemodynamic monitoring specialist disconnects the arterial and pulmonary pressure lines, if present, and transfers the lines to the transport monitor, balancing the transducers. When the patient is completely connected to the transport monitor, the patient can be disconnected from the unit's monitoring system. If an intra-aortic balloon is in place, the EKG electrodes connected to the balloon pump are not removed so that the patient's hemodynamic status can be monitored off of the balloon pump screen.	The patient's hemodynamics are continuously monitored. Invasive pressure lines must be recalibrated when changing monitors to maintain accurate pressure readings.
6. The circulating nurse ensures that the patient is transported with supplemental oxygen in place, if ordered. The anesthesiologist is present if the patient is being mechanically ventilated.	Supplemental oxygen is given to augment the patient's own oxygen reserve. The anesthesiologist is responsible for maintaining the airway with adequate ventilation.
7. The patient is transferred to surgery in the unit bed and to the operating table by the transporters.	Exertion increases the oxygen demand on the heart.
8. The patient is connected to the noninvasive monitors, EKG, BP, and pulse oximeter in the surgical suite. The transport leads are disconnected and removed. The invasive lines are disconnected from the transport monitor and connected to the transducers and monitor in the surgical suite. EKG leads connected to a balloon pump are left in place and a slaving cable is connected to the monitor in the surgical suite.	The patient's hemodynamics are continuously monitored. The slaving cable adapts the EKG tracing from the balloon pump to the monitor in the surgical suite.

Steps:	Rationale:
9. The circulating nurse pads and tucks the patient's arms at his or her sides.	Allows access to the surgical field. Bony prominences are protected.
10. The surgical table safety strap is applied over the patient's thighs.	Helps prevent the patient from rolling off the bed.
11. The surgeons are notified.	Facilitates the surgical process.

Standard of Care: Cardiac Surgery: Transfer of the Unstable Cardiac Patient to Surgery

I. Priorities of Care
   A. Interdepartmental communication
      1. Facilitates the perioperative plan of care
   B. Expedite the surgical process
      1. Time is life—seconds count
      2. Coordinated team response
      3. Safe and efficient transfer of the patient from the unit to surgery
II. Interdepartmental Communication Between the Patient Care Unit and Surgery
   A. Current patient physiologic status is reported to the circulator
      1. Physical assessment
      2. Invasive lines, type and location
      3. Cardiac supportive drugs
      4. Any mechanical assist devices
         a. IABP
         b. LVAD/RVAD/CPS
         c. Pacemaker, internal defibrillator
         d. Ventilator dependent
   B. Circulating nurse communicates transfer time to the unit nurse
      1. Surgical consent is obtained.
      2. Blood is typed and cross-matched.
      3. Surgical shave prep is completed.
      4. If time allows, a bladder Foley catheter is inserted.
      5. The circulating nurse and the hemodynamic monitoring technician assist in the transfer of the patient from the unit to surgery. The anesthesiologist assists in the transport if the patient is ventilator dependent.
      6. The patient is properly identified. The pre-op checklist is completed, and the nursing physical assessment is accomplished.
      7. The hemodynamic monitoring specialist transfers the patient EKG cables and the arterial and PA pressure lines to the transfer monitor. If the intra-aortic balloon is in place, the balloon pump can be used to monitor the patient.
      8. Supplemental oxygen is given, per physician order.
      9. Communication with family members is completed.
      10. The patient is transferred to the operating room in the unit bed.

III. The Patient Is Transferred to the Surgical Table
   A. The monitoring equipment is transferred from the transport monitor to the surgical suite monitoring equipment.
   B. The unit bed is sent back to the unit.
   C. The anesthesiologist and surgeons are present.
   D. Noninvasive monitoring devices are applied.
   E. The patient's arms are padded and tucked at his or her sides.
   F. The table strap is applied over the patient's legs.
   G. Emergency equipment is available and functioning should the need arise.
   H. Preparation is made for the surgical prep. Bladder Foley catheter is inserted, if not previously done, and blood is sent from the blood bank as soon as it becomes available.
   I. All attempts are made to expedite the surgical process.
IV. Clinical Indicators for Evaluation
   A. Preoperative assessment
      1. Perioperative plan of care consistent with the needs of the patient
      2. Interdepartmental communication to meet the patient's needs
      3. Safe transfer of the patient to the surgical suite
      4. Surgical expediency and preparedness
   B. Patient outcome

Cardiac Surgery: Policy: Surgical Shave Prep for Cardiac Surgical Procedures

Cardiac surgery's policy is that all patients undergoing a cardiac surgical procedure require removal of hair at the incision site(s) before surgery, meeting the following criteria:

1. Physician order for a shave prep
2. The shave prep is done according to the written protocol for the specific cardiac surgical procedure.
3. The shave prep is completed as close to the surgical procedure as possible.
4. The shave prep is done with a hair clipper only. Razors are not used.

Cardiac Surgery: Nursing Procedure: Shave Prep for Valve Replacement/Repair Procedures

Quality Outcome: Safe and effective removal of hair surrounding the incision site(s) is performed to facilitate optimum exposure, preventing inadvertent skin breakdown, with risk of infection.

Performed by: Registered nurses, orderlies, and nursing assistants

General Statement: Patients undergoing valve replacement/repair procedures have the hair removed from the following area:
  A. Chest—the patient is shaved from the neck to the umbilicus, approximately 10 inches wide, nipple line to nipple line. It is not necessary to shave the chest of a woman.
  B. Perineal area—the entire perineal area is shaved.
  C. Legs—the femoral areas, along with the anterior to medial side of the thighs, to the knees, are shaved.

Equipment: Hair clipper, disposable shaving heads for the clipper, and nonsterile gloves

Steps:	Rationale:
1. The chart is checked for the physician's order for a shave prep. The patient is properly identified, and the shave prep is explained.	The surgeon is responsible for designating the need for hair removal. Explaining the procedure, with the rationale, will alleviate anxiety related to the procedure.
2. Privacy during the shave prep is provided. The area to be shaved is draped to expose only the area to be shaved.	Skin preparation can be an embarrassing procedure for the patient. Draping off the area to be shaved prevents unnecessary exposure.
3. The integrity of the skin is documented before the hair is removed.	Abnormal skin irritation, infection, or abrasion on or near the operative site might be a contraindication to an operation.
4. Good illumination is provided.	Permits adequate lighting for hair removal.

Steps:	Rationale:
5. Unsterile gloves are put on, and a disposable razor head is inserted into the clipper.	Gloves are worn to prevent cross-contamination. Clippers cut hair close to the skin.
6. The chest is shaved first, followed by the legs and perineal area.	The areas considered clean are shaved first followed by the areas considered less clean.
7. After the shave prep is completed, the area(s) shaved is documented. The name of the individual performing the shave prep is documented.	All care, along with the person shaved and the condition of the skin, is documented.
8. The razor head is disposed of properly and the clipper is cleaned according to hospital policy.	The clipper head is cleaned and disinfected to prevent cross-contamination.

Cardiac Surgery: Nursing Procedure: Shave Prep for Cardiothoracic Surgical Procedures

Quality Outcome: Safe and effective removal of hair surrounding the incision site(s) is performed to facilitate optimum exposure, preventing inadvertent skin breakdown, with risk of infection.

Performed by: Registered nurses, orderlies, and nursing assistants

General Statement: Patients undergoing cardiothoracic surgical procedures have the hair removed from the following areas:

- A. Chest—the chart is checked for verification of the correct surgical site, left or right chest. The patient's chest is shaved from the shoulder to the umbilicus, bed line to bed line. It is not necessary to shave the chest of a woman.
- B. Perineal area—the entire perineal area is shaved.
- C. Legs—the femoral areas, along with the anterior side of the thighs, to the knees, are shaved. The femoral arteries must be accessible for these procedures for cardiopulmonary bypass and/or intra-aortic balloon insertion.

Equipment: Hair clipper, disposable shaving heads for the clipper, and nonsterile gloves

Steps:	Rationale:
1. The chart is checked for the physician's order for a shave prep. The correct surgical side, left or right chest, is verified. The patient is properly identified, and the shave prep is explained.	The surgeon is responsible for designating the need for hair removal. Explaining the procedure, with the rationale, will alleviate anxiety related to the procedure.
2. Privacy during the shave prep is provided. The area to be shaved is draped to expose only the area to be shaved.	Skin preparation can be an embarrassing procedure for the patient. Draping off the area to be shaved prevents unnecessary exposure.
3. The integrity of the skin is documented before the hair is removed.	Abnormal skin irritation, infection, or abrasion on or near the operative site might be a contraindication to an operation.

Steps:	Rationale:
4. Good illumination is provided.	Permits adequate lighting for hair removal.
5. Unsterile gloves are put on, and a disposable razor head is inserted into the clipper.	Gloves are worn to prevent cross-contamination. Clippers cut hair close to the skin.
6. The patient is placed in a lateral position to facilitate the shaving of the chest.	Cardiothoracic procedures require a lateral chest incision site. The areas considered clean are shaved first.
7. The patient is then positioned supine to shave the perineal area and anterior thighs to the knees.	Provides better exposure for further shaving.
8. After the shave prep is completed, the area(s) shaved is documented. The name of the individual performing the shave prep is documented.	All care, along with the person shaved and the condition of the skin, is documented.
9. The razor head is disposed of properly, and the clipper is cleaned according to hospital policy.	The clipper head is cleaned and disinfected to prevent cross-contamination.

Cardiac Surgery: Nursing Procedure: Shave Prep for CABG Surgical Procedures

Quality Outcome: Safe and effective removal of hair surrounding the incision site(s) is performed to facilitate optimum exposure, preventing inadvertent skin breakdown, with risk of infection.

Performed by: Registered nurses, orderlies, and nursing assistants

General Statement: Patients undergoing coronary artery bypass procedures have the hair removed from the following areas:
  A. Chest—the patient is shaved from the neck to the umbilicus, approximately 10 inches wide, nipple to nipple. It is not necessary to shave the chest of a woman.
  B. Perineal area—the entire perineal area is shaved.
  C. Legs—the medial aspects of both legs are shaved from the groin to the ankles.

Equipment: Hair clipper, disposable shaving heads for the clipper, and nonsterile gloves

Steps:	Rationale:
1. The chart is checked for the physician's order for a shave prep. The patient is properly identified and the shave prep is explained.	The surgeon is responsible for designating the need for hair removal. Explaining the procedure, with the rationale, will alleviate anxiety related to the procedure.
2. Privacy during the shave prep is provided. The area to be shaved is draped to expose only the area to be shaved.	Skin preparation can be an embarrassing procedure for the patient. Draping off the area to be shaved prevents unnecessary exposure.
3. The integrity of the skin is documented before the hair is removed.	Abnormal skin irritation, infection, or abrasion on or near the operative site might be a contraindication to an operation.
4. Good illumination is provided.	Permits adequate lighting for hair removal.

Steps:	Rationale:
5. Unsterile gloves are put on, and a disposable razor head is inserted into the clipper.	Gloves are worn to prevent cross-contamination. Clippers cut hair close to the skin.
6. The chest is shaved first, followed by the legs and perineal area.	The areas considered clean are shaved first, followed by the areas considered less clean.
7. After the shave prep is completed, the areas rendering the care are documented. The name of the individual performing the shave prep is documented.	All care, along with the person shaved and the condition of the skin, is documented.
8. The razor head is disposed of properly and the clipper is cleaned according to hospital policy.	The clipper head is cleaned and disinfected to prevent cross-contamination.

Standard of Care: Cardiac Surgery: Cardiac Surgical Shave Preps

I. Indications for Hair Removal
   A. Surgeon's orders
   B. Hair that interferes with exposure
   C. Hair that interferes with closure
   D. Hair that interferes with dispersive electrode pad placement and adherence
   E. Hair that interferes with EKG electrode pad placement
II. Special Considerations Regarding Shave Preps
   A. The patient is informed of the procedure.
      1. The patient's privacy is maintained.
   B. Shave preps are completed as close to the surgical time as possible.
   C. The condition of the patient's skin is assessed.
   D. Preps are completed with a clipper or depilatory cream.
III. Cardiac Surgical Shave Preps
   A. CABS
      1. Anterior chest, neck to umbilicus
      2. Perineal area
      3. Lower extremities
   B. Valve procedures
      1. Anterior chest, neck to umbilicus
      2. Perineal area
      3. Lower extremities to the knees
   C. Cardiothoracic procedures
      1. Left posterolateral chest
      2. Perineal area
      3. Lower extremities to the knees
IV. Documentation
   A. Type of shave prep performed
   B. Assessment of the skin before and after the shave prep
   C. The name of the person completing the shave prep
   D. The date and time of the shave prep
V. Clinical Indicators for Evaluation
   A. Efficacy and effectiveness of the surgical shave prep
   B. Infection rate
   C. Condition of the patient's skin, preoperatively

Cardiac Surgery: Policy: Continual Quality Improvement

Cardiac surgery's policy is to monitor routine activities, document variances, audit clinical outcomes, and conduct problem-focused studies to assess actual practices and evaluate outcomes of patient care. This established quality improvement program provides systematic monitoring and evaluation of, but is not limited to, the following:

1. Patient care activities
2. Case management
3. Scheduling
4. Staffing
5. Continuing education
6. Environmental precautions
7. Risk management
8. Fiscal management

Standard of Care: Cardiac Surgery: Total Quality Management

I. Goals of Continual Quality Management
    A. Monitor the appropriateness of patient care
    B. Evaluate the quality of patient care
    C. Resolve identified problems
        1. Identify areas for improvement
        2. Improve
    D. Establish clinical indicators as tools for evaluation

II. Indicators
    A. Patient care activities
    B. Events
    C. Occurrences
    D. Outcomes

III. Components of Total Quality Management
    A. Administrative
        1. Attainable goals
        2. Fiscal management
            a. Case management
                1. Inventory of supplies
                2. Inventory of instrumentation
                3. Inventory of equipment
                4. Time management
        3. Medical–legal aspects
            a. Policies
            b. Procedures
            c. Standards of care
            d. Regulatory compliance
        4. Staff development
            a. Definition of individual roles
            b. Education
                1. Specific educational requirements
                    a. CPR certified
                    b. ACLS certified
                    c. Continuing education
        5. Staff meetings
        6. Performance reviews
        7. Skills checklist
        8. Networking
        9. Orientation process

- a. Orientation manual
- b. Standards of care
10. Preceptor
    - a. Orientation evaluation
11. Nursing research

B. Communication
   1. Scheduling
      - a. Elective
      - b. Emergent
      - c. Urgent
   2. Call coverage
   3. Computer access
      - a. Record keeping
      - b. Utilization review

C. Environmental precautions
   1. Housekeeping protocols
   2. Infection control

D. Risk management
   1. Universal precautions
      - a. Personal protective equipment
   2. Safety
      - a. Electrical safety
      - b. Staff safety
      - c. Patient safety
   3. Variance documentation and evaluation

E. Facility
   1. Accessibility to the surgical suite
   2. Room preparation

F. Patient Care
   1. Nursing care plan
      - a. Assessment
      - b. Planning
      - c. Implementation
      - d. Evaluation
   2. Reassessment to meet the needs of the patient
   3. Policies and procedures
   4. Standards of care
   5. Documentation

Intraoperative Management

chapter 8

Cardiac Surgery: Policy: Physiologic Monitoring for Cardiac Surgical Procedures

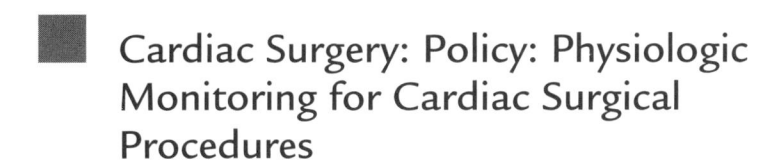

Cardiac surgery's policy is that physiologic monitoring of a patient undergoing a cardiac/cardiothoracic surgical procedure consists of noninvasive and invasive techniques to indicate minute-to-minute changes in the physiologic variables. These surgical patients are monitored continuously.

Noninvasive monitoring is to include but is not limited to the following:

1. Cardiac monitoring using a five-lead EKG.
2. Peripheral blood pressure with appropriate-size blood pressure cuff.
3. Oxygen saturation using a pulse oximeter.
4. Esophageal stethoscope for monitoring body temperature.
5. Entropy sensor for monitoring patient's level of consciousness

Invasive monitoring is to include but is not limited to the following:

1. Arterial and venous pressures
    a. Arterial line/transducer
    b. Swan-Ganz catheter/transducer
        1. CVP; measure volume
        2. Cardiac output
        3. SVO_2
2. Renal function
    a. Foley catheter

3. Physiologic lab values
    a. Hematocrit
    b. ACT/HPT
    c. Electrolytes
    d. Acid–base values
    e. Oxygen saturation, venous and arterial blood

Cardiac Surgery: Nursing Procedure: Physiologic Monitoring for Cardiac Surgical Procedures

Quality Outcome: Physiologic monitoring detects minute-to-minute changes in the hemodynamic status of the patient, allowing the team to assess, interpret, respond to, and evaluate the therapy instituted.

Performed by: Cardiac anesthesiologist, circulating nurse, and hemodynamic monitoring specialist

General Statement: The patient's hemodynamics are continuously monitored intraoperatively and postoperatively using invasive and noninvasive monitoring techniques.

Equipment: Blood pressure cuff/automatic blood pressure monitor, pulse oximeter finger probe/monitor, five-lead EKG cable/electrodes, tape, entropy sensor, arterial and venous transducers/cables, arterial catheters, Swan-Ganz/CVP catheters, cardiac output monitor, and SVO_2 monitor

Steps:	Rationale:
1. After positioning the patient on the surgical table, the circulating nurse and the hemodynamic monitoring specialist position the noninvasive monitoring equipment. The EKG electrodes are placed one on each arm, one on each hip, laterally, and one on the lateral chest wall, making sure that there is good skin contact. Hair is removed if necessary. Tape is placed over the electrodes.	The position of the electrodes is dependent on optimal surgical exposure permitting well-defined cardiac monitoring. Electrodes do not adhere well to hair. Tape is used to prevent dislodgement of the electrodes intraoperatively.
2. The blood pressure cuff is placed on the opposite arm of the invasive arterial line.	This prevents occlusion of the arterial line and allows continuous monitoring without interruption.
3. The pulse oximeter probe is placed on a finger.	Permits monitoring of oxygen saturation.
4. The safety strap is applied over the patient's thighs.	Facilitates patient safety on a narrow surgical table by inhibiting leg movements.

Steps:

5. The hemodynamic monitoring specialist organizes the equipment needed for invasive line placement and assists the anesthesiologist as needed. The circulating nurse observes the patient and monitors for changes in the hemodynamic status. Emergency equipment is available.

6. Postoperatively, the patient is transferred to the intensive care unit with cardiac and arterial pressure monitoring.

Rationale:

Assistance may be needed with invasive line placement. Ventricular irritability may occur during placement of invasive lines.

Continual monitoring is accomplished to monitor changes in the patient's physiologic status.

Standard of Care: Cardiac Surgery: Physiologic Monitoring

I. Types of Physiologic Monitoring During a Cardiac Procedure
   A. The patient is continually monitored
      1. Noninvasive monitoring
      2. Invasive monitoring
II. Noninvasive Monitoring
   A. Five-lead EKG
   B. Blood pressure
      1. The blood pressure cuff is placed on an arm, unless contraindicated, on the side opposite the arterial line placement.
      2. The blood pressure cuff is appropriate for the size of the extremity.
   C. Oxyhemoglobin
      1. Pulse oximeter
         a. Finger probe or ear probe
   D. Temperature
      1. Esophageal stethoscope
      2. Rectal probe, if indicated by the type of myocardial protection
      3. Bladder temperature catheter
III. Invasive Monitoring
   A. Arterial pressure
      1. Sites that can be used
         a. Radial artery
         b. Brachial artery
         c. Femoral artery
   B. Central venous pressure
      1. CVP
   C. Left ventricular pressures
      1. Sites that can be used
         a. Left or right internal jugular vein
         b. Left or right subclavian vein
         c. Left or right femoral vein
      2. Pressure measurements
         a. Pulmonary artery pressures
            1. PAD pressures
            2. PCWP pressures
      3. Cardiac output
      4. Mixed venous saturation
      5. SVR
   D. Urine output

      E. Physiologic lab values
IV. Documentation of Physiologic Monitoring
      A. Documented on the following records
          1. Surgical record
          2. Anesthesia record
          3. Perfusion record
          4. ICU documentation record
      B. Documentation specifics
          1. Type of monitoring equipment used
          2. Sites of invasive line placement
          3. Type and size of catheters used
          4. Name of person inserting the invasive lines
          5. Medications given
V. Clinical Indicators for Evaluation
      A. Staff education pertaining to physiologic monitoring
          1. Indications
          2. Normal ranges
          3. Perioperative plan of care dependent on the patient's current physiologic values
          4. Assistance to the anesthesiologist with physiologic monitoring placement
              a. Time needed to implement noninvasive and invasive physiologic monitoring
      B. Availability of the physiologic monitoring equipment
      C. Evaluation of the level of monitoring required
      D. Infection rate associated with the invasive line placement
      E. The method by which the invasive lines are secured to prevent dislodgement
      F. Complete documentation

Cardiac Surgery: Policy: Blood Utilization

Cardiac surgery's policy is that

1. Patients sign an informed transfusion consent indicating their approval for, or refusal of, transfusions, should the need arise.
2. Bank blood is available before the start of the surgical procedure and is stored near the cardiac surgical suite in a temperature-monitored blood refrigerator or an ice cooler with a temperature-sensing indicator bag for the duration of the cardiac surgical procedure.
3. Staff members handling blood must wear protective gloves.
4. Blood is not removed from the temperature-controlled environment until it is to be used.
5. Blood units are checked between two licensed individuals according to hospital policy.
6. Designated donor units are used before universal donor units.
7. Blood that expires first is used first.
8. All transfusions are documented on the surgical record, the fluid flow sheet, and the transfusion record.
9. Any indications of a transfusion reaction are documented, and appropriate action is taken.
10. Empty blood bags are placed in a protective, sealed bag and returned to the blood bank.
11. Bank blood is returned to the blood bank after the patient has been transferred to the intensive care unit.

Cardiac Surgery: Nursing Procedure: Bank Blood Acquisition

Quality Outcome: Blood is available and properly identified before the start of the cardiac surgical procedure.
Performed by: Circulating nurse and nursing assistant
General Statement: Bank blood is available for cardiac surgery, unless refused by the patient, and is stored near the cardiac surgical suite.
    The blood is stored, until needed, in a temperature-monitored blood refrigerator or ice cooler with a temperature-indicator bag for the duration of the cardiac surgical procedure.
Equipment: Blood refrigerator or an ice cooler with a temperature-sensing indicator

Steps:	Rationale:

1. Preoperatively, the circulating nurse checks the chart for the following:
  a. Transfusion consent
  b. Blood has been typed and crossed.
  c. A blood identification band is located on the patient's wrist.
	Bank blood is available for every cardiac surgical procedure unless refused by the patient.

2. Prior to induction, the circulating nurse completes the required documentation to transfer the blood from the blood bank to the surgical suite.
This includes but is not limited to
  a. The patient's name and date
  b. Blood identification number
  c. Type and amount of blood products requested
	Blood bank requirements are completed.

Steps:	Rationale:
3. A nursing assistant is called to the surgical suite to retrieve the blood from the blood bank. The appropriate documentation accompanies the assistant to the blood bank.	Blood products are obtained from the blood bank and released to a responsible person after verification of the patient in comparison with the blood.
4. The blood bank is called and informed that the blood is to be retrieved.	Facilitates the transfer without unnecessary delays.
5. After the surgical procedure and after the patient has been transferred to the unit, the blood is returned to the blood bank.	Blood is available for the postoperative period.

Standard of Care: Cardiac Surgery: Blood Utilization

I. Initial Preparation
   A. An informed consent is required for the use of universal blood/blood products.
      1. A refusal to accept blood or blood products consent is signed, if applicable.
   B. A predetermined amount of blood is typed and cross-matched within 48–72 hours of the surgical procedure and is available the day of surgery.
      1. Designated donor blood
      2. Universal bank blood
II. Intraoperative Blood Storage and Handling
   A. Bank blood or designated donor blood is procured from the blood bank before the cardiac surgical procedure begins.
   B. The blood is stored until needed, in the following, dependent on hospital policy
      1. A temperature-regulated and monitored blood refrigerator
      2. An ice cooler with a temperature-sensing control indicator
   C. Protective gloves are worn when handling blood products.
   D. Empty blood bags are placed in sealed bags and returned to the blood bank.
   E. Unused blood is returned to the blood bank as soon as the patient is transferred to the intensive care unit.
III. Intraoperative Blood Utilization
   A. Bank blood is properly identified, per hospital policy, before the case begins and before each time the patient is transfused.
   B. The cell saver and the heart–lung machine aid in blood return.
   C. Blood-soaked sponges are gently squeezed out before discarding, recovering the blood with the use of the cell saver or cardiotomy suction line.
   D. Designated donor blood is used first, if available, followed by universal donor blood, as the need arises. The blood units that are closer to the expiration date are used first.
   E. A specified amount of available blood, per surgeon request, is kept ahead, if transfusing multiple units.
   F. All unit identification numbers, type, and amount of blood given are documented on the operative record and fluid flow sheet.
   G. Time of transfusion and end of transfusion along with the patient's reaction to the transfusion are documented on the transfusion record.
   H. The names of the staff members checking the blood and giving the blood are documented on the transfusion record.

IV. Intraoperative Blood Salvaging Techniques
   A. Autologous
      1. Cell saver; primary conduit for blood salvaging intraoperatively, before heparinization and after cardiopulmonary bypass with protamine reversal.
      2. Cardiopulmonary bypass cardiotomy suction; primary conduit for blood salvaging used after heparinization for cardiopulmonary bypass.
      3. Cardiopulmonary bypass vent line; accessory suction line capable of returning intraoperative shed blood to the heart–lung machine after heparinization.
   B. Heart–lung machine
      1. Capable of returning large amounts of fluid/blood products quickly to the patient through the cardiopulmonary bypass circuits
   C. Hemoconcentration
      1. Remaining blood volume in the heart–lung oxygenator is filtered to remove plasma.
      2. The red blood cells are concentrated and returned to the patient at high hematocrit levels.
V. Postoperative Blood Salvaging
   A. Pleural drainage unit collects the shed mediastinal fluid, filters it, and returns it to the patient.
VI. Quality Indicators for Evaluation
   A. Blood availability
      1. Blood bank typed and crossed at the appropriate time
      2. Time involved retrieving the blood/blood products from the blood bank
      3. Evaluating supply of blood products versus demand
   B. Decreased need for bank blood intraoperatively
      1. Intraoperative surgical technique
      2. Tracking and recognizing trends in type and amounts of blood/blood products that are given intraoperatively
   C. The patient's hemodynamic stability
      1. Hematocrit
         a. Preoperative, intraoperative, and postoperative
      2. Arterial and venous oxygen saturation
      3. Heart rate and blood pressure
      4. Activated clotting time
   D. Reactions to transfusion
      1. Type
      2. Incidence

Cardiac Surgery: Policy: Autotransfusion

Cardiac surgery's policy is that autotransfusion using a cell-saver machine will be available for every cardiac surgical procedure.

The operation of the cell-saver machine will be performed by a licensed individual meeting the following requirements but not limited to the following:

A. Licensed individual trained and oriented by the manufacturer or perfusion provider.
B. Proctored on a minimum of 10 cases
C. Perfusionist

Cardiac Surgery: Nursing Procedure: Autotransfusion

Quality Outcome: Autologous, intraoperative shed blood is collected, processed, and washed, reinfusing the packed cells to the patient.

Performed by: Perfusionist and licensed individual, meeting the operational requirements

General Statement: Autotransfusion is available for elective and emergent cardiac and cardiothoracic surgical procedures.

Equipment: Autotransfusion machine, suction regulator, sterile aspiration set, autotransfusion pack, collection reservoir, normal saline, injectable fluid bags, 1000 ml, heparin, 10,000 units per ml of saline

Steps:	Rationale:
1. The autotransfusion pack and the collection reservoir are assembled on the autotransfusion machine by the licensed operator.	The autotransfusion pack is assembled according to manufacturer's instructions.
2. The collection reservoir is connected to 120- to 150-mm Hg regulated suction.	Vacuum must be regulated to decrease the lysis of red cells.
3. Normal saline, 1000 ml, is hung on the autotransfusion machine with 30,000 units of heparin additive.	Heparinized saline prevents clotting of the shed blood in the aspiration conduit from the field to the autotransfusion reservoir.
4. The sterile aspiration set is opened for the scrub nurse.	This set is the conduit from the field to the autotransfusion collection reservoir.
5. The scrub nurse passes off two ends of the aspiration conduit to the circulating nurse.	The aspiration conduit consists of a dual lumen. One lumen is a conduit for shed blood; the other is a spiked conduit for the heparinized saline to prevent the blood from clotting en route to the autotransfusion reservoir.

Steps:	Rationale:
6. The circulating nurse connects one end of the aspirating tubing from the field to the collection reservoir and the spiked end to the heparinized solution, setting the heparinized saline at a slow, continuous drip. The suction conduit is always connected to the reservoir first, verifying suction.	After the aspiration conduit is connected to the autotransfusion machine, aspiration and collection of shed blood are possible. Heparinized saline will spill over the sterile field if the suction is not working or is connected after the heparinized saline conduit has been connected.
7. The scrub nurse uses the cell saver as the primary aspiration conduit until the patient is heparinized and placed on cardiopulmonary bypass and used again after cessation of cardiopulmonary bypass with protamine reversal.	After cardiopulmonary bypass is initiated, the cardiotomy aspiration conduit connected to the heart–lung machine is used, directing blood back to the heart–lung machine.
8. Processing of the collected blood is initiated after the volume of blood collected in the reservoir has reached 500 to 800 ml.	It takes 500 to 600 ml of volume to fill the centrifugal bowl on the autotransfusion machine.
9. The blood in the collection reservoir is spun down into the spinning centrifugal bowl. After the bowl is completely filled, its contents are washed with a liter of normal saline.	Excess fluid is spun off and discarded, separating the plasma from the red cells. The saline wash removes the heparin from the red blood cells.
10. When the wash cycle is completed, the bowl is stopped and the red blood cells are returned to a transfusion pack and given to the patient.	The processing is complete and the cells are ready to return to the patient.
11. The transfusion pack is labeled with the patient name and given to the anesthesiologist.	The unit to be infused is properly identified.

Steps:	Rationale:
12. The total volume reinfused to the patient is documented.	Facilitates evaluation of volume needs of the patient.
13. After the patient is transferred to the intensive care unit, the autotransfusion system is broken down and discarded appropriately. Protective gloves are worn. The machine is cleaned with a disinfectant.	The risk of cross-contamination is decreased by observing the proper precautions.

Cardiac Surgery: Policy: Stat Lab Protocol

Cardiac surgery's policy is that the following criteria be maintained by the department of perfusion regarding the cardiac surgery stat lab but are not limited to

1. Written and updated policies and procedures pertinent to the stat lab
2. Maintenance of CLIA and state licensure
    a. Lab determinations are completed by the perfusionist.
    b. Performance of the required quality assurance checks on the lab equipment
    c. Required documentation of quality assurance checks and routine maintenance of lab equipment

Cardiac Surgery: Nursing Procedure: Maintenance of the Stat Lab

Quality Outcome: The safe use of the stat lab in the cardiac surgical suite is accomplished by performing the required quality assurance checks, maintenance, and documentation required to maintain CLIA and state licensure.

Performed by: Perfusionist, and physicians or staff demonstrating competency

General Statement: The perfusionist's responsibility is to follow and maintain the requirements mandated by CLIA and the state.

Equipment: Stat lab equipment, quality lab check cartridges for the individual pieces of equipment, and log.

Steps:	Rationale:
1. The perfusionist is responsible for the composition of the procedures for each specific lab determination completed within the surgical suite. These procedures follow the specific guidelines set up by the manufacturers and are reviewed and revised annually.	Complies with JCAHO state and federal regulations.
2. The procedure for the quality assurance checks on each piece of lab equipment is performed before the start of each case by the perfusionist.	All equipment is checked before the start of the surgical procedure to prevent unnecessary surgical delays. The stat labs' test results are compared with the quality assurance tests run and the guidelines provided by the manufacturer.
3. The perfusionist records the quality assurance test results from each piece of lab equipment and stores the information in a log book or computer for future reference. The manufacturers' name along with the model and serial numbers of the equipment utilized are documented.	Documentation of the quality assurance process is required by CLIA and state regulations to maintain stat lab licensure.

Steps:	Rationale:
4. If a discrepancy arises on a piece of lab equipment, all further tests are sent to the main hospital laboratory until the equipment can be checked and repaired. The perfusionist coordinates the repair of the equipment with the manufacturer. The equipment is cleaned before shipment.	Lab determinations during cardiac surgery facilitate the intraoperative care of the patient. The surgeon is dependent on accurate information in order to treat the patient appropriately. Any equipment leaving the hospital must be cleaned according to OSHA guidelines.
5. Routine maintenance is performed on all stat lab equipment. Maintenance records are maintained for future reference.	Stat lab equipment is safe and functioning at all times for elective or emergent cases.
6. Any new stat lab equipment or loaner equipment must be checked with the biomedical department before use.	Required safety checks are completed before use.

Standard of Care: Cardiac Surgery: Stat Lab

I. Cardiac Surgical Stat Lab Capability
   A. Arterial and venous blood gases
   B. Electrolytes
   C. Hematocrit
   D. Activated clotting time (ACT)
   E. Heparin dose response (HDR)
   F. Heparin protamine titration (HPT)
   G. Glucose
II. Quality Control Program
   A. Blood Gas QC
      1. Two levels of quality control—one at the beginning of each 8-hr period of use and one level during the 8-hr period or according to manufacturer's instructions and hospital policy.
   B. Electrolytes QC
      1. Two levels of quality control—one at the beginning of each 8-hr period of use and one level during the 8-hr period or according to manufacturer's instructions and hospital policy.
   C. Hematocrit QC
      1. Two levels of quality control at the beginning of each 8-hr period of use or according to manufacturer's instructions and hospital policy.
   D. ACT QC
      1. One level of quality control at the beginning of each 8-hr period of use or according to manufacturer's instructions and hospital policy.
   E. HDR QC
      1. Performed according to manufacturer's instructions and hospital policy.
   F. HPT QC
      1. One level of quality control at the beginning of each 8-hr period of use for each cartridge type used or according to manufacturer's instructions and facility policy.
   G. Glucose QC
      1. Two levels of quality control at the beginning of each 8-hr period of use or according to manufacturer's instructions and facility policy.
III. Proficiency Testing Program
   A. CLIA requires moderate test lab equipment to be enrolled in a proficiency testing program.

- B. Tests for HPT and HDR are to follow the specific stat lab manufacturers' recommendations.
- C. Glucose is an excluded test.
IV. Lab Licensure
- A. All stat labs must be licensed by OSSIFY and in some cases the state.
- B. To maintain licensure
    1. Only perfusionists or physicians or licensed personnel that demonstrate competency annually may perform tests.
    2. A standard operating procedure must be established and followed.
    3. Quality control results are kept with the lab equipment.
    4. Proficiency tests must be performed and passed.
V. Preventive Maintenance
- A. Equipment should be kept clean and free of bodily fluids.
- B. Biannual electrical safety checks must be performed.
- C. The manufacturer's recommended preventive maintenance schedule must be maintained.
VI. Clinical Indicators for Evaluation
- A. Quality control program is monitored.
    1. Reliability of the lab equipment
- B. Maintenance of licensure
- C. Cost of supplies and testing

Cardiac Surgery: Policy: Surgical Skin Prep for Cardiac Surgical Procedures

Cardiac surgery's policy is that patients undergoing a cardiac surgical procedure be prepped with an approved broad-spectrum antimicrobial solution according to the specific cardiac surgical procedure to be performed.

The patient's history is checked for allergies before the surgical scrub procedure.

Time out for the surgical scrub to dry is provided and documented.

■ Cardiac Surgery: Nursing Procedure: Surgical Skin Prep for Valve Procedures

Quality Outcome: Resident microorganisms are reduced by mechanical and chemical cleansing of the skin with an approved broad-spectrum antimicrobial solution.

Performed by: Circulating nurse

General Statement: After the patient is induced and positioned, the circulating nurse preps the patient from the neck to the knees. Time is permitted prior to incision to permit the prepping solution to dry and time from initial prep and incision is documented.

Equipment: Sterile prep tray, sterile gloves, and broad-spectrum antimicrobial solution

Steps:

1. After the patient is positioned, the circulating nurse prepares the prep tray. The circulating nurse checks the patient's history of allergies and assesses the patient's skin.

2. The antimicrobial solution is warmed if the patient is to be prepped awake.

3. The circulating nurse preps the patient from the neck to the knees.

Rationale:

The history of allergies is checked before application of the antimicrobial solution to decrease the chance of an allergic reaction. The integrity of the skin is assessed to prevent the possibilities of an untoward reaction to the surgical prep.

Unstable cardiac patients may be prepped and draped awake to save valuable time should an arrest occur during induction. The warmed antimicrobial solution aids in temperature loss and provides comfort to the patient.

The complete operative site and periphery are prepped. The femoral areas need to be prepped and exposed should cardiopulmonary bypass be implemented through the femoral arteries or an intra-aortic balloon inserted.

Steps:	Rationale:
4. The circulating nurse ensures that the antimicrobial solution does not pool under the patient. Time is permitted for prepping solution to dry, and time is documented.	Pooling of the antimicrobial solution can cause skin irritation and chemical burns. Time is allowed for the prepping solution to dry to provide safe patient care with the use of electrocautery.
5. The circulating nurse assesses the patient's reaction to the prep solution. If a skin reaction occurs, the prep is discontinued, an alternative solution is used, and the surgeon is notified.	Assessment of the skin during and after the prepping procedure prevents the chance of complications.

6. Documentation of the surgical prep includes, but is not limited to
  a. Preoperative condition of the skin
  b. Type of antimicrobial solution used
  c. Site prepped
  d. Name of the nurse completing the prep
  e. Patient's reaction to the surgical prep
  f. Time out procedure indicating prepping drying time prior to incision.
	All details of the skin condition and skin preparation are documented. Time out for the prepping solution to dry provides additional safety measures with the use of electrocautery.

Cardiac Surgery: Nursing Procedure: Surgical Skin Prep for Cardiothoracic Procedures

Quality Outcome: Resident microorganisms are reduced by mechanical and chemical cleansing of the skin with an approved broad-spectrum antimicrobial solution.

Performed by: Circulating nurse

General Statement: After the patient is induced and positioned, the circulating nurse preps the patient from the left shoulder, tableside to tableside on the chest, extending to the knees. Time is permitted prior to incision to permit the prepping solution to dry, and time from initial prep and incision is documented.

Equipment: Sterile prep tray, sterile gloves, and broad-spectrum antimicrobial solution

Steps:	Rationale:
1. After the patient is positioned, the circulating nurse prepares the prep tray. The circulating nurse checks the patient's history of allergies and assesses the patient's skin.	The history of allergies is checked before application of the antimicrobial solution to decrease the chance of an allergic reaction. The integrity of the skin is assessed to prevent the possibilities of an untoward reaction to the surgical prep.
2. The antimicrobial solution is warmed if the patient is to be prepped awake.	Unstable cardiac patients may be prepped and draped awake to save valuable time should an arrest occur during induction. The warmed antimicrobial solution aids in temperature loss and provides comfort to the patient.
3. The circulating nurse preps the patient from the left shoulder to the knees and from table side to table side on the chest.	The complete operative site and periphery are prepped. The femoral areas need to be prepped and exposed should cardiopulmonary bypass be implemented through the femoral arteries.

Steps:	Rationale:
4. The circulating nurse ensures that the antimicrobial solution does not pool under the patient. Time is permitted for prepping solution to dry, and time is documented.	Pooling of the antimicrobial solution can cause skin irritation and chemical burns. Time out for the prepping solution to dry provides additional safety measures with the use of electrocautery.
5. The circulating nurse assesses the patient's reaction to the prep solution. If a skin reaction occurs, the prep is discontinued. An alternative solution is used, and the surgeon is notified.	Assessment of the skin during and after the prepping procedure prevents the chance of complications.

6. Documentation of the surgical prep includes but is not limited to
  a. Preoperative condition of the skin
  b. Type of antimicrobial solution used
  c. Site prepped
  d. Name of the nurse completing the prep
  e. Patient's reaction to the surgical prep
  f. Time out procedure indicating prepping drying time prior to incision.
	All details of the skin condition and skin preparation are documented. Time out for the prepping solution to dry provides additional safety measures with the use of electrocautery.

Nursing Procedure: Surgical Skin Prep for Cardiothoracic Procedures

Cardiac Surgery: Nursing Procedure: Surgical Skin Prep for CABG Procedures

Quality Outcome: Resident microorganisms are reduced by mechanical and chemical cleansing of the skin with an approved broad-spectrum antimicrobial solution.

Performed by: Circulating nurse

General Statement: Two circulating nurses are required to complete the CABG surgical skin prep, one on each side of the patient.

After the patient is induced and positioned, the circulating nurses prep the patient from the neck to the toes bilaterally and around the entire circumference of the legs.

Equipment: Sterile prep tray, sterile gloves, and broad-spectrum antimicrobial solution

Steps:	Rationale:
1. After the patient is positioned, the circulating nurse prepares the prep trays. The circulating nurse checks the patient's history of allergies and assesses the patient's skin.	The history of allergies is checked before application of the antimicrobial solution to decrease the chance of an allergic reaction. The integrity of the skin is assessed to prevent the possibilities of an untoward reaction to the surgical prep.
2. The antimicrobial solution is warmed if the patient is to be prepped awake.	Unstable cardiac patients may be prepped and draped awake to save valuable time should an arrest occur during induction. The warmed antimicrobial solution aids in avoiding temperature loss and provides comfort to the patient.
3. This prep requires two circulating nurses to prep the patient, one on each side of the patient. The patient is prepped from the neck to the toes bilaterally. The circumference of the legs is prepped.	The complete operative site and periphery are prepped. The lower extremities are prepped and exposed for saphenous vein harvesting. The surgical skin prep is completed quickly and efficiently with two circulating nurses.

4. The circulating nurse ensures that the antimicrobial solution does not pool under the patient.

Pooling of the antimicrobial solution can cause skin irritation and chemical burns.

5. The circulating nurse assesses the patient's reaction to the prep solution. If a skin reaction occurs, the prep is discontinued. An alternative solution is used, and the surgeon is notified.

Assessment of the skin during and after the prepping procedure prevents the chance of complications.

6. Documentation of the surgical prep includes but is not limited to
   a. Preoperative condition of the skin
   b. Type of antimicrobial solution used
   c. Site prepped
   d. Names of the nurses completing the prep
   e. Patient's reaction to the surgical prep
   f. Time out procedure indicating prepping drying time prior to incision.

All details of the skin condition and skin preparation are documented. Time out for the prepping solution to dry provides additional safety measures with the use of electrocautery.

Standard of Care: Cardiac Surgery: Cardiac Surgical Skin Preps

I. Criteria for Surgical Skin Preps
   A. Procedure to be performed
   B. Surgical approach
   C. The patient's history of allergies
   D. Surgeon preference
   E. Preoperative condition of the skin
II. Safety Measures
   A. Patient
      1. The history of allergies is verified preoperatively.
      2. The skin is assessed preoperatively.
      3. The antimicrobial prep solution is not permitted to pool beneath the patient.
      4. Time is provided for the prepping solution to dry and is documented.
III. Criteria for Prep Solutions
   A. Broad-spectrum antimicrobial action
   B. Quickly applied and remains effective on the skin
   C. Nonflammable
   D. Nontoxic
IV. Cardiac Surgical Skin Preps
   A. CABG
      1. Requires two circulating nurses, one on each side of the patient
         a. The patient is prepped from the neck to the toes bilaterally, starting at the chest and working down toward the feet.
         b. The circumference of both lower extremities is prepped.
            1. Vein harvesting procedure
   B. Valve procedures
      1. Requires only one circulating nurse
         a. The patient is prepped from the neck to the knees bilaterally.
            1. The femoral area must be prepped in case femoral cannulation or an intra-aortic balloon pump is needed.
   C. Cardiothoracic procedures
      1. Requires one circulating nurse
      2. Prepped from the left shoulder to the knees
         a. The femoral area must be prepped in case femoral cannulation or an intra-aortic balloon pump is needed.
V. Documentation
   A. Preoperative condition of the skin
   B. Type of antimicrobial solution used

      C. Site prepped
      D. Name of the nurse(s) completing the prep
      E. Patient's reaction to the surgical skin prep
      F. Time out performed to allow surgical prepping solution to dry and documented
VI. Clinical Indicators for Evaluation
      A. Nursing assessments
          1. Condition of the patient's skin
          2. Safety precautions
      B. Nursing interventions
      C. Effectiveness of the surgical prep
          a. Infection control
      D. Patient's response to treatment

Cardiac Surgery: Policy: Positioning for Cardiothoracic Surgical Procedures

Cardiac surgery's policy is that the lateral position be used for cardiothoracic procedures to provide optimum exposure and access to the surgical site. The following criteria must be assessed to assure proper body alignment and maintain tissue integrity.

1. The patient's physical condition
2. Anatomical and physiologic considerations
3. Left or right lateral position
   a. Accessibility to the femoral arteries and veins for extracorporeal circulation, if warranted
4. Safety and security measures
5. Patient monitoring
6. Documentation of position and positioning devices used

Cardiac Surgery: Nursing Procedure: Positioning for Cardiothoracic Surgical Procedures

Quality Outcome: Optimal surgical exposure is provided while maintaining the patient's proper body alignment and tissue integrity intraoperatively.

Performed by: Circulating nurse, anesthesiologist, and ancillary personnel

General Statement: The patient's lateral position should provide access to the surgical site as well as the patient's airway, intravenous lines, and monitoring devices. The position does not compromise integumentary, circulatory, respiratory, musculoskeletal, or neurological structures.

Equipment: Bean bag, pillows, axillary rolls, foam padding, arm board/over-the-bed arm support, tape, and safety belt

Steps:	Rationale:
1. Preoperatively, the circulating nurse assesses the patient's special needs, including physical limitations, weight, height, nutritional status, skin condition, preexisting disease, and type and length of procedure.	Drugs or anesthetic agents can alter the patient's existing physical limitations. Adipose tissue is not well perfused. Underweight patients experience pressure on bony prominences. Malnourished patients are at greater risk for tissue damage. Hypothermia, hypotension, and prolonged length of procedures without a position change can lead to decreased tissue perfusion. Unperfused tissue has an increased risk for pressure ulcers.
2. The circulating nurse verifies the correct surgical position and organizes the appropriate positioning equipment required. Bean bag, pillows, axillary rolls, foam padding, and tape are available nearby.	Position for the operation is determined by the procedure to be performed, with consideration of the surgeon's surgical approach and the patient's physical condition.

Steps:	Rationale:
3. The bean bag is positioned under a draw sheet on the surgical table prior to the patient's transfer and is to be under the patient's torso. The bean bag is tested by applying vacuum to ensure that it will stay firm.	The bean bag stabilizes the patient's torso. All equipment is tested before use to ensure patient safety and to keep anesthesia and surgical time to a minimum.
4. The patient is transferred to the surgical table after induction. A safety strap is applied over the patient's thighs.	The patient is positioned initially in a supine position. The safety strap inhibits leg movements.
5. During induction, the circulating nurse coordinates the number of personnel to adequately position the patient.	Sufficient personnel and slowly positioning the patient contribute to patient and personnel safety.
6. The patient is turned on his or her unaffected side, operative side up. The bottom leg is padded and flexed, and the top leg is straight. Pillows are placed between the two legs. Ankles are padded. The upper arm is placed on a raised armboard, if available. If a conventional armboard is used, pillows are used to place between the arms. The femoral arteries and veins must be accessible.	This position provides access to the underlying ribs and widens the intercostal spaces. Exposure to the femoral arteries and veins is necessary for extracorporeal circulation should femoral–femoral bypass be instituted.
7. An axilla roll is placed at the apex of the scapula.	The lower shoulder is brought slightly forward to prevent pressure on the brachial plexus and allows greater chest movement with respirations.
8. Vacuum is applied to the bean bag.	Vacuum makes the bean bag firm and supports the weight and position of the patient.

Steps:	Rationale:
9. Tape is applied over the patient's shoulder and hips and is connected to the surgical table. A blanket is placed over the lower portion of the patient.	Tape is added for additional support. Undue exposure may lower body temperature and should be limited to preserve patient dignity.

10. After positioning, the circulating nurse assesses the patient's body alignment and tissue integrity. The assessment includes but is not limited to
   a. Respiratory
   b. Musculoskeletal
   c. Circulatory
   d. Neurological
   e. Integumentary
	Positions can influence respirations by mechanically restricting the rib cage and abdomen. Anesthetic agents cause dilation of peripheral blood vessels with a drop in blood pressure. Improper positioning on the surgical table can cause postoperative palsies.

11. The dispersive electrode pad is positioned.	Necessary for safe electrocautery use

12. The following is documented on the operative record:
   a. Position
   b. Positional devices
   c. Protective devices, type, and site
   d. Safety restraints
   e. Any adverse effects related to the surgical position
	Intraoperative care is documented.

Positioning for Valve Replacement/Repair Policy
Unit: Cardiac Surgery: Nursing Procedure

It is cardiac surgery policy that patient's scheduled for valve replacement/repair procedures be placed in a supine position, arms padded and tucked at the side, and a rolled towel be placed under the shoulders. The head is supported with a head rest to prevent hyperextension of the neck.

The lower extremities are slightly everted to provide exposure to the femoral arteries, should the need arise for femoral-femoral cannulation for cardiopulmonary bypass or an intra-aortic balloon catheter.

Quality Outcome: The patient is positioned for safety and surgical accessibility for the valvular replacement or repair procedure along with exposure to the femoral arteries should the need arise.

Performed by: Cardiac anesthesiologist and circulating nurses.

General Statement: The patient is positioned on the surgical table, supine, arms placed at the sides so that neck to knees is exposed for surgical access. The circulating nurse assesses the patient to see whether the patient is able to move to the surgical table on his or her own or needs assistance due to an underlying physical disability or the current cardiovascular status.

Equipment: Ulnar nerve pads, padded roll towels, and birdcage if available.

Steps:	Rationale:
1. Preoperatively, the circulating nurse assesses the patient's special needs, including physical limitations, weight, height, nutritional status, skin condition, preexisting disease, and type and length of the surgical procedure. If the patient is extremely short of breath, the patient is assisted to the surgical table with a roller. A pillow is placed under the patient's head or the head of the bed is raised.	Drugs or anesthetic agents can alter the patient's existing physical limitations. Adipose tissue is not well perfused. Underweight patients experience pressure on bony prominences. Malnourished patients are at a much higher risk for tissue damage. Hypothermia, hypotension, and prolonged length of the procedure can lead to decreased tissue perfusion. Under-perfused tissue has an increased risk for pressure ulcers. Valve patients present in different stages of congested failure. Raising the head of the patient facilitates the work of breathing and makes the patient more comfortable.

Steps:	Rationale:
2. The patient is positioned supine on the surgical table after transfer from the gurney/bed. The patient's arms are placed on arm boards until the invasive lines have been inserted. During induction, the arms are placed at the patient's sides with protective ulnar nerve pads covering the elbows. A safety strap is applied over the thighs. The dispersive electrode pad is positioned.	The supine position facilitates the access for invasive line placement and optimum exposure for the institution of cardiopulmonary bypass and revascularization of the heart. The ulnar pads prevent pressure points with damage to the ulnar nerve. The safety strap inhibits leg movements. The dispersive electrode pad is necessary for safe electrocautery use.
3. A padded roll is placed under the shoulders of the patient.	The padded roll raises the level of the chest and extends the neck to facilitate the surgical access at the sternal notch.
4. After the Swan-Ganz line is inserted, if applicable, the birdcage or mayo stand is positioned over the head of the patient. The patient's gown and blankets are removed.	The birdcage or mayo stand can be used as an overhead table for aspiration lines, internal paddles, and saw. The birdcage/mayo stand also protects the patient's head during surgery. The blankets are not removed until the circulating nurse is ready to prep the patient to preserve body heat and maintain the privacy of the patient.
5. The circulating nurse slightly frog legs the patient's lower extremities before the surgical prep.	The legs are slightly frogged for access to the femoral arteries should the need to cannulate the arteries for cardiopulmonary bypass or insertion of an intra-aortic balloon pump become necessary.
6. If the surgeon is doing a CABG/valve replacement/repair procedure, the positioning for CABG procedures is followed.	The necessary exposure for the surgical procedure is provided.

Steps:	Rationale:
7. After positioning, the circulating nurse assesses the patient's body alignment and tissue integrity. This assessment includes but is not limited to the following: a. Respiratory b. Musculoskeletal c. Circulatory d. Neurological e. Integumentary	Anesthetic agents cause dilation of peripheral blood vessels with a drop in blood pressure. Improper positioning on the surgical table can cause postoperative palsies.
8. The following is documented on the operative report: a. Position b. Positional devices c. Protective devices d. Any adverse effects related to the surgical position	All intraoperative care is documented.

Cardiac Surgery: Policy: Positioning for CABG Procedures

Cardiac surgery's policy is that a patient scheduled for CABG procedures be placed in the supine position, arms padded and tucked at the sides, and a rolled towel be placed under the shoulders. The head is supported with a headrest to prevent hyperextension of the neck.

Both lower extremities are slightly everted to provide exposure for

1. Saphenous vein and or radial artery harvesting
2. Access to the femoral arteries, should the need arise for femoral–femoral cannulation for cardiopulmonary bypass or insertion of an intra-aortic balloon catheter

The patient is positioned for optimum surgical exposure and safety.

The position and positioning devices used are documented on the surgical record.

Cardiac Surgery: Nursing Procedure: Positioning for CABG Procedures

Quality Outcome: The patient is positioned for safety and surgical accessibility for the revascularization process and vein-harvesting procedure.
Performed by: Cardiac anesthesiologist and circulating nurses.
General Statement: The patient is positioned on the surgical table, supine, arms placed at the sides so that the neck to the toes is exposed for surgical access. The circulating nurse assesses the patient to see whether the patient is able to move to the surgical table on his or her own or needs assistance because of an underlying physical disability or the current cardiovascular status.
Equipment: Ulnar nerve pads, padded roll, towels, and birdcage, if available.

Steps:	Rationale:
1. Preoperatively, the circulating nurse assesses the patient's special needs, including physical limitations, weight, height, nutritional status, skin condition, preexisting disease, and type and length of the surgical procedure. The cardiovascular status of the patient is assessed prior to the transfer of the patient to the table. If chest pain develops while the patient is moving to the surgical table, the patient is assisted with a roller.	Drugs or anesthetic agents can alter the patient's existing physical limitations. Adipose tissue is not well perfused. Underweight patients experience pressure on bony prominences. Malnourished patients are at a much higher risk for tissue damage. Hypothermia, hypotension, and prolonged length of the procedure can lead to decreased tissue perfusion. Underperfused tissue has an increased risk for pressure ulcers. Physical exertion causes an increase in oxygen demand on the heart. Patients scheduled for revascularization of the myocardium may not tolerate the increase in myocardial workload caused by the increase in oxygen demands.

Steps:	Rationale:
2. The patient is positioned supine on the surgical table after transfer from the gurney/bed. The patient's arms are placed on arm boards until the invasive lines have been inserted. During induction, the arms are placed at the patient's sides with protective ulnar nerve pads covering the elbows. A safety strap is applied over the thighs.	The supine position facilitates the access for invasive line placement and optimum exposure for the institution of cardiopulmonary bypass and revascularization of the heart. The ulnar pads prevent pressure points with damage to the ulnar nerve. The safety strap inhibits leg movements.
3. A padded roll is placed under the shoulders of the patient. The dispersive electrode pads are placed.	The padded roll raises the level of the chest and extends the neck to facilitate the surgical access at the sternal notch. The dispersive pads are necessary for safe electrocautery use.
4. After the Swan-Ganz line is inserted, if applicable, the birdcage or mayo stand is positioned over the head of the patient. The patient's gown and blankets are removed.	The birdcage or mayo stand can be used as an overhead table for aspiration lines, internal paddles, and saw. The birdcage/mayo stand also protects the patient's head during surgery. The blankets are not removed until the circulating nurse is ready to prep the patient to preserve body heat and maintain the privacy of the patient.
5. A leg holder is positioned over the lower half of the surgical table in preparation of the surgical prep. The legs are not placed up in the holder until it is time to prep.	The leg holder facilitates the circumferential prep of the legs. The patient's legs are not placed in the holder until it is time to prep because the raised legs cause an increase in venous return to the heart, and some cardiac patients cannot tolerate this sudden increase in blood flow.

Steps:	Rationale:
6. The circulating nurse removes the legs from the holder, prepping the feet. The legs are held in the air until the scrub nurse positions the sterile drapes on both legs from the feet to the femoral region. After the table has been draped, the circulating nurse lowers the legs onto the sterile drapes.	The legs are draped out completely to permit exposure to the saphenous veins on both legs from the feet to the femoral region. The lesser saphenous vein on the posterior side of the leg may be used if the saphenous veins have been used or are not good quality for vascular conduits.
7. The scrub nurse places the legs in a frog position with rolled towels under the knees. After positioning, the circulating nurse and scrub nurse assesses the patient's body alignment and tissue integrity. This assessment includes but is not limited to 　a. Respiratory 　b. Musculoskeletal 　c. Circulatory 　d. Neurological 　e. Integumentary	The frog-leg position facilitates the vein-harvesting procedure. The rolled towels are placed under the knees for support. Anesthetic agents cause dilation of peripheral blood vessels with a drop in blood pressure. Improper positioning on the surgical table can cause postoperative palsies.
8. The following is documented on the operative report: 　a. Position 　b. Positional devices 　c. Protective devices, type, and size 　d. Any adverse effects related to the surgical position.	All intraoperative care is documented.

Standard of Care: Cardiac Surgery: Positioning for Cardiac Surgical Procedure

I. Criteria for Positioning
   A. Procedure to be performed
   B. Surgical approach
   C. Preoperative assessment of the patient for positioning needs
      1. Physical limitations
      2. Weight
      3. Nutritional status
      4. Skin condition
      5. Preexisting disease
      6. Type and length of procedure
      7. Positional devices needed
II. Safety Measures
   A. Patient
      1. Maintenance of proper body alignment
         a. Anatomical and physiological considerations
            1. Respiratory
            2. Circulation
            3. Musculoskeletal
            4. Neurological
            5. Integumentary
      2. Maintenance of tissue integrity
         a. Padding for pressure points
         b. Padded positional devices
   B. Staff
      1. Sufficient personnel to lift, turn, or transfer the patient
III. Cardiac Procedures
   A. CABG
      1. Supine
      2. Lower extremities slightly everted, knees supported
      3. Arms padded and tucked at the side
      4. Padded roll under the shoulders
      5. Safety strap over thighs, preoperative and postoperative
   B. Valve procedures
      1. Supine
      2. Lower extremities slightly everted
      3. Arms padded and tucked at the sides

        4. Padded roll under the shoulders
        5. Safety strap over the thighs
        6. Blanket over the lower extremities
    C. Cardiothoracic
        1. Lateral
            a. Left
            b. Right
            c. Bean bag
            d. Femoral artery access
            e. Pillows between the legs
            f. Foam pads under the lower ankle and knee
            g. Arm boards
            h. Axillary rolls under arms
            i. Tape over the shoulder and hip
            j. Safety strap over the thighs
            k. Blanket over the lower extremities

IV. Documentation
    A. Positioning
    B. Type and placement of positioning equipment
    C. Positional changes made during the procedure
    D. Padding devices
    E. Safety straps
    F. Patient's response to positioning

V. Quality Indicators for Evaluation
    A. Positioning devices are available and tested for the specific procedure
    B. Patient is free of injury at the completion of the procedure
    C. Historical clinical data derived from medical documentation for analysis and review
        1. Care given
        2. Nursing assessments
        3. Nursing interventions
        4. Patient's response

Cardiac Surgery: Policy: Draping for the Cardiac Surgical Procedure

Cardiac surgery's policy is that standards of care for draping be established to facilitate the surgical process, meeting the following criteria but not limited to

1. Creates and maintains a sterile field
2. Provide optimal exposure to the surgical sites
3. Can be easily and quickly applied
4. Meets the requirements of AORN standards

Cardiac Surgery: Nursing Procedure: Draping for a Valve Replacement/Valve Repair Procedure

Quality Outcome: A sterile barrier is created for a valve replacement/valve repair procedure, allowing optimum access to the surgical incision site.

Performed by: Cardiac surgeon and scrub nurse

General Statement: The anterior chest, abdomen, and inguinal areas are exposed for surgical access during the valve replacement/valve repair procedures

Equipment: Cardiovascular fenestrated drape, extra-large antimicrobial-impregnated plastic incise drape, and sterile towels

Steps:	Rationale:
1. The scrub nurse opens the appropriate supplies needed for draping.	All supplies needed for draping are opened and available to prevent unnecessary intraoperative delays.
2. The scrub nurse organizes the draping material on a ring stand in the order to be used. The ring stand and drapes are pulled close to the surgical table to facilitate the draping process. The scrub nurse stands on the opposite side of the table while assisting the surgeon with the draping process.	Drapes are organized on a ring stand so that they can be pulled to either side of the surgical table. The draping process must be accomplished quickly and efficiently to meet the needs of the changing hemodynamic status of the patient.

Steps:

3. Draping the anterior chest: The scrub nurse hands the surgeon four folded towels to drape off the anterior chest.
   a. A towel is placed above the sternal notch.
   b. A towel is placed across the abdomen at the level of the umbilicus.
   c. A towel is run along both sides of the chest at the nipple line, connecting the towels at the top and bottom
   d. A towel is used to blot the exposed skin.
   e. A towel is folded in thirds and placed over the perineum.
   f. The femoral area is isolated with towels, leaving the femoral artery sites exposed.
   g. The extra-large antimicrobial-impregnated incise drape is spread out over the toweled-off area, extending from the sternal notch to the inguinal area.
   h. The cardiovascular fenestrated sheet is spread out over the entire patient, starting at the head of the patient, extending down the sides of the surgical table towards the feet.

4. A fan-folded drape sheet is spread out over the legs, extending towards the feet.

Rationale:

The four towels are positioned to isolate the area for the chest incision. A dry towel is used to blot off the excess prep solution so that the plastic incise drape will adhere to the skin. Plastic incise drapes alleviate the need for towel clips and aid in preventing the migration of normal skin flora into the surgical wound. The perineum is covered to decrease the chance of wound contamination. The femoral arteries are accessible in case an intra-aortic balloon needs to be inserted or femoral bypass instituted. The cardiovascular fenestrated sheet provides a sterile field with the use of only one drape. It also has pockets capable of securing the extracorporeal circuits in place during the procedure.

The legs are covered to prevent cross-contamination from the legs to the chest.

Cardiac Surgery: Nursing Procedure: Draping for the Coronary Artery Bypass Procedure

Quality Outcome: A sterile barrier is created for a coronary artery bypass procedure, allowing optimum access to the surgical incision sites.

Performed by: Cardiac surgeon and scrub nurse

General Statement: The anterior chest, abdomen, and legs are exposed for surgical access during the coronary artery bypass procedure.

Equipment: Cardiovascular fenestrated drape, fan-folded drape sheet, plastic "U" drape, extra-large antimicrobial-impregnated plastic incise drape, and sterile towels

Steps:

1. The scrub nurse opens the appropriate supplies needed for draping.

2. The scrub nurse organizes the draping material on a ring stand in the order to be used. The ring stand and drapes are pulled close to the surgical table to facilitate the draping process. The scrub nurse stands on the opposite side of the table while assisting the surgeon with the draping process.

Rationale:

All supplies needed for draping are opened and available to prevent unnecessary intraoperative delays.

Drapes are organized on a ring stand so that they can be pulled to either side of the surgical table. The draping process must be accomplished quickly and efficiently to meet the changing hemodynamic status of the patient.

Steps:

3. The legs are left exposed for saphenous vein harvesting. The circulating nurse preps both legs, circumferentially. The circulating nurse holds the legs until the scrub nurse places the sterile drape sheets under the legs. Drapes for the lower extremities are as follows:
   a. A plastic "U" drape is placed under the legs pulling the lower portion of the drape over the end of the surgical table, then extending the "U" portion of the drapes along each side of the surgical table extending towards the patient's head.
   b. A fan-folded drape is spread out over the plastic "U" drape.
   c. A towel, folded in thirds, is placed over the perineum.
   d. The legs are lowered onto the sterile drapes, and a stockinette is placed over both feet, extending to the ankles.

Rationale:

The search for good saphenous veins used for coronary grafting can incorporate the use of one or two legs and can include the lesser saphenous vein on the posterior aspect of the legs, depending on the integrity of vein and the amount of vein needed. A sterile barrier is achieved by placing sterile drapes under the legs or arms. The feet, hands and perineum are covered to decrease the chance of wound contamination.

Steps:	Rationale:

4. Draping the anterior chest: The scrub nurse hands the surgeon four folded towels to drape off the anterior chest.
   a. A towel is placed above the sternal notch.
   b. A towel is placed across the abdomen at the level of the umbilicus.
   c. A towel is run along both sides of the chest at the nipple line, connecting the towels at the top and bottom.
   d. A towel is used to blot the exposed skin.
   e. The extra-large antimicrobial-impregnated incise drape is spread out over the toweled-off area, extending from the sternal notch to the inguinal area.
   f. The cardiovascular fenestrated sheet is spread out over the entire patient, starting at the head of the patient, extending down the sides of the surgical table toward the feet.
	The four towels are positioned to isolate the area for the chest incision. A dry towel is used to blot off the excess prep solution so that the plastic incise drape will adhere to the skin. Plastic incise drapes alleviate the need for towel clips and aid in preventing the migration of normal skin flora into the surgical wound. The cardiovascular fenestrated sheet provides a sterile field with the use of only one drape. It also has pockets capable of securing the extracorporeal circuits in place during the procedure.

5. When the saphenous vein harvesting is completed, a fan-folded drape sheet is placed over the legs by the scrub nurse.	The legs are covered to prevent cross-contamination from the legs to the chest.

Cardiac Surgery: Nursing Procedure: Draping for a Cardiothoracic Surgical Procedure

Quality Outcome: A sterile barrier is created for a cardiothoracic procedure, allowing optimum access to the surgical incision sites.

Performed by: Cardiac surgeon and scrub nurse

General Statement: The anterior and posterior portions of the chest to the knees are exposed for surgical access during the cardiothoracic procedure.

Equipment: Cardiovascular fenestrated drape, extra-large antimicrobial-impregnated plastic incise drape, and sterile towels

Steps:	Rationale:
1. The scrub nurse opens the appropriate supplies needed for draping.	All supplies needed for draping are opened and available to prevent unnecessary intraoperative delays.
2. The scrub nurse organizes the draping material on a ring stand in the order to be used. The ring stand and drapes are pulled close to the surgical table to facilitate the draping process. The scrub nurse stands on the opposite side of the table while assisting the surgeon with the draping process.	Drapes are organized on a ring stand so that they can be pulled to either side of the surgical table. The draping process must be accomplished quickly and efficiently to meet the needs of the changing hemodynamic status of the patient.

Steps:	Rationale:

3. Draping the chest anteriorly and posteriorly: The scrub nurse hands the surgeon four folded towels to drape off the anterior chest.
   a. A towel is placed across the shoulder.
   b. A towel is placed across the abdomen, anteriorly and posteriorly at the level of the umbilicus.
   c. A towel is run along both sides of the chest at the bed line, connecting the towels at the top and bottom.
   d. A towel is used to blot the exposed skin.
   e. A towel is folded in thirds and placed over the perineum.
   f. The femoral area is isolated with towels, leaving the femoral artery sites exposed.
   g. The extra-large antimicrobial-impregnated incise drape is spread out over the toweled-off area, extending from the sternal notch to the inguinal area.
   h. The cardiovascular fenestrated sheet is spread out over the entire patient, starting at the head of the patient, extending down the sides of the surgical table toward the feet.
	The four towels are positioned to isolate the area for the chest incision. A dry towel is used to blot off the excess prep solution so that the plastic incise drape will adhere to the skin. Plastic incise drapes alleviate the need for towel clips and aid in preventing the migration of normal skin flora into the surgical wound. The perineum is covered to decrease the chance of wound contamination. The femoral arteries are accessible in case an intra-aortic balloon needs to be inserted. The cardiovascular fenestrated sheet provides a sterile field with the use of only one drape. It also has pockets capable of securing the extracorporeal circuits in place during the procedure.

4. The legs are covered.	The legs are covered to prevent cross-contamination from the legs to the chest.

Standard of Care: Cardiac Surgery: Draping for the Cardiac Surgical Procedure

I. Indications for an Aseptic Barrier
   A. Creation of a sterile field
   B. Maintenance of a sterile field
   C. Prevention of wound contamination
II. Criteria for Draping Materials
   A. Resistant to liquid penetration
   B. Resistant to tears and punctures
   C. Lint free
   D. Materials meet or exceed the standards of the National Fire Protection Association
   E. Contours to the patient's body easily
   F. Can be easily and quickly applied
III. Positioning of the Surgical Drapes
   A. Dependent on the type of surgical procedure performed
      1. Optimal exposure to the surgical site is provided
   B. The femoral region is draped out and accessible for all cardiac and cardiothoracic surgical procedures.
   C. Completed after the surgical prep
   D. Completed by the surgeon and scrub nurse
IV. Draping for a Coronary Bypass Procedure
   A. Accessible areas
      1. Anterior chest
         a. Towels are positioned to drape off the sternal area.
            1. A towel folded in half is placed above the sternal notch.
            2. A towel folded in thirds is placed across the abdomen at the umbilicus.
            3. A towel folded in half is placed at the breast line bilaterally.
      2. Femoral region
         a. A towel folded in thirds is placed over the perineum, extending to the towel over the umbilicus.
      3. A large plastic incise drape sheet impregnated with iodine is placed over all of the towels.
      4. The lower extremities
         a. A drape sheet is placed under the legs while the circulating nurse is finishing the last of the prep.
         b. The legs are lowered onto the sterile drape.

    c. Sterile towels are placed under the knees to facilitate the saphenous vein harvesting.
    d. A sterile towel or stockinette is placed over both of the feet.
    e. If the arm is used, a sterile drape is placed under the arm, a towel folded in thirds is placed around the upper arm, and an extremity drape is applied. A towel is placed over the fingers, palm side up, to facilitate position for the radial artery harvesting.
   5. A large fenestrated cardiovascular split sheet is positioned over the entire patient.
    a. A barrier is created between anesthesia and the sterile field
    b. The sides of the drape are run along both sides of the patient and positioned on the sides of the bed from the neck to the toes.
V. Draping for a Valve Replacement/Repair Procedure
 A. Accessible areas
  1. Anterior chest
   a. Towels are positioned to drape off the sternal area.
    1. A towel folded in half is placed above the sternal notch.
    2. A towel folded in thirds is placed across the abdomen at the umbilicus.
    3. A towel folded in half is placed at the breast line bilaterally.
  2. Femoral region
   a. A towel folded in thirds is placed over the perineum, extending to the towel over the umbilicus.
   b. The femoral region is isolated with towels from the umbilicus to the knees bilaterally.
 B. A large plastic incise drape sheet impregnated with iodine is placed over all of the towels.
 C. A paper drape sheet is placed over the legs from the knees extending toward the feet.
 D. A large fenestrated cardiovascular split sheet is positioned over the entire patient.
  1. A barrier is created between anesthesia and the sterile field.
  2. The sides of the drape are run along both sides of the patient and positioned on the sides of the bed from the neck to the toes.
VI. Draping for a Cardiothoracic Surgical Procedure
 A. Accessible areas
  1. Left or right lateral chest dependent on the specific cardiovascular procedure performed
   a. Towels are placed around the surgical incision site, extending from the breast to the middle portion of the back.
    1. A folded towel is placed across the shoulder.
    2. A folded towel is placed across the hip.

3. A folded towel is placed at the table side of the patient on both sides, joining the towels positioned at the top and bottom of the patient.
      2. The femoral region is isolated with towels from the umbilicus to the knees bilaterally.
   B. A large plastic incise drape sheet impregnated with iodine is placed over all the towels.
   C. A paper drape sheet is placed over the legs from the knees extending toward the feet.
   D. A large fenestrated cardiovascular split sheet is positioned over the entire patient.
      1. A barrier is created between anesthesia and the sterile field
      2. The sides of the drape are run along both sides of the patient and positioned on the sides of the bed from the neck to the toes.
VII. Clinical Indicators for Evaluation
   A. Effectiveness of the sterile barrier
   B. Infection control
   C. Ease of application
   D. Meets AORN standards

Cardiac Surgery: Policy: Cardiopulmonary Bypass

Cardiac surgery's policy is that the following guidelines be established for cardiopulmonary bypass, including but not limited to

1. Cardiopulmonary bypass is instituted under the direction and supervision of the cardiac surgeon.
2. The perfusionist is responsible for the preparation, maintenance, and discontinuation of cardiopulmonary bypass.
3. Cardiopulmonary bypass is not initiated until systemic heparinization of the patient is completed with acceptable ACT and HPT level determinations achieved.
4. A perfusion protocol is written and followed.
5. Accurate documentation of cardiopulmonary bypass is completed.
6. Evaluation of the patient's response to cardiopulmonary bypass is followed.
7. Maintenance of the heart–lung machine is the responsibility of the perfusionist and is done according to the manufacturer's guidelines and as deemed necessary.

Introduction to Cardiopulmonary Bypass and Myocardial Protection

A quiet, motionless heart and bloodless operative field are desirable for a portion of time during myocardial revascularization and valvular repairs and/or replacements. Myocardial energy resources are preserved by manually arresting the heart during cardiopulmonary bypass, lowering the systemic temperature, and cooling the heart.

This necessitates the use of extracorporeal circulation via the heart–lung machine. The heart–lung machine functions as the patient's own heart and lungs, continually providing adequate cardiac output and proficient organ perfusion during the cardiac surgical procedure. The metabolic needs of the heart are decreased dramatically by lowering the patient's systemic body temperature by cooling the blood returning to the heart–lung machine and topical cooling with cold irrigation or slush.

The blood is circulated from the patient to the heart–lung machine through a closed circuit of four different tubings, each with a different destination and function.

The circuit areas follow:

A. Cardioplegia line: This line infuses cardioplegia, which chemically arrests the heart and provides the necessary nutrients to the myocardium while on cardiopulmonary bypass. This line is filled with cold or warm crystalloid or blood perfusate, dependent on the surgeon preference and type of procedure, after initiation of cardiopulmonary bypass and connected to the antegrade and/or retrograde cardioplegia catheter for delivery.
B. Cardiotomy suction: This conduit is used to return shed operative blood back to the reservoir on the heart–lung machine after systemic heparinization has been instituted.
C. Vent circuit: This circuit is connected to the aortic root cannula or a left pulmonary vein vent catheter with low suction applied to help facilitate a "bloodless" field. During massive hemorrhage, this circuit can be used as an additional cardiotomy suction to facilitate the return of blood to the reservoir on the heart–lung machine.
D. A–V loop: This circuit starts out as one continuous line, but after it is primed with crystalloid solution or blood from the pump and the line is completely free of air, it is divided by the scrub nurse/tech. The smaller of the conduits becomes the arterial line, returning oxygenated blood from the pump to the patient. The larger circuit becomes the venous return line, directing deoxygenated blood from the right atrium to the heart–lung machine to be oxygenated.

Anticoagulation therapy is instituted before extracorporeal circulation to inhibit clot formation within the pump circuit. The dose of heparin is dependent on the patient's weight. Heparin is given by the surgeon via the right atrium or by the anesthesiologist before cardiopulmonary bypass. The perfusionist performs ACT tests at regular intervals while on bypass and gives additional heparin as necessary to prevent coagulation. Protamine is given after bypass is discontinued to counteract the heparin.

During cardiopulmonary bypass, the blood is circulated at a speed that maintains all hemodynamic parameters; oxygen and carbon dioxide are exchanged, and the blood temperature is regulated.

The heart–lung machine has the capacity to deliver large amounts of fluids, blood, and drugs if necessary.

Cannulation of the femoral artery and vein is performed when there is an urgent need to place the patient on bypass and CPR is being initiated; redo cardiac surgical procedures when the chest cannot be entered quickly and CPR is in progress or the aorta is extremely calcified. Femoral cannulation is the site of choice when dealing with ascending and descending thoracic aortic aneurysms.

After cardiopulmonary bypass has been instituted, the patient's body temperature is lowered, and the cardioplegia is delivered to provide the necessary nutrients to the myocardium. Slush may be placed in the pericardium. Cardioplegia is delivered at timed intervals to maintain arrest and nutrient stores. Dependent upon the procedure and the surgeon, a normothermic state may be chosen versus lowering the patient's body temperature. If the patient is kept normalthermic, slush is exchanged for warm saline irrigation. After the surgical revascularization or valve repair/replacement is completed, and before discontinuation of cardiopulmonary bypass, the patient's systemic temperature is increased to normal body temperature. Any remaining slush is removed. The ability to wean a patient successfully from cardiopulmonary bypass requires hemostasis and hemodynamic stability. This includes adequate circulating blood volume and filling pressures, good cardiac rhythm and output, normothermia, and no signs of hemorrhage from the multiple surgical sites. The high concentrations of potassium used in the cardioplegia solution are reversed using insulin. If a patient is hypothermic, myocardial irritability will ensue. After these parameters are met, the cardiopulmonary bypass circuits are removed. The pump circuits are removed from the field and discarded when the patient is stabilized and the sternal wires are in place.

Cardiac Surgery: Nursing Procedure: Institution of Cardiopulmonary Bypass

Quality Outcome: Cardiopulmonary bypass is initiated quickly and efficiently without any complications.

Performed by: Cardiac surgeon, cardiac anesthesiologist, perfusionist, hemodynamic monitoring specialist, circulating nurse, and scrub nurse

General Statement: All team members are educated in the process of cardiopulmonary bypass with individualized roles coordinated to expedite the procedure safely.

Equipment: Extracorporeal table circuit, venous perfusion cannula, arterial perfusion cannula, heart–lung machine, cannulation stitches, tourniquets, and heparin

Steps:	Rationale:
1. The scrub nurse opens the extracorporeal table circuit on to the sterile field. Perfusion cannulas and cannulation stitches are gathered and opened. All tubing and cannulation stitches are prepared in advance.	It is the scrub nurse's responsibility to open all supplies needed for the procedure before scrubbing. Perfusion equipment and cannulation stitches are prepared early in anticipation of an emergency.
2. During the initial case preparation, the perfusionist prepares the heart–lung machine and completes the prebypass safety checks. The heparin dose is calculated, and the prebypass lab determinations are completed.	The perfusionist must be available with the pump primed when the surgeon opens the chest to be prepared if the patient's condition deteriorates, requiring rapid sternotomy, cannulation, and cardiopulmonary bypass. The heparin dose is determined by the weight of the patient and/or the heparin dose response test.
3. The circulating nurse sends for the bank blood and checks it with the perfusionist if it is needed to prime the pump.	The nurse assures that blood products are available, checked, and ready for immediate use. Anticipation for blood utilization can be expected if the patient's hematocrit is low.

Steps:	Rationale:
4. All members of the team are constantly aware of the patient's hemodynamic status to detect changes that would require quick, organized responses.	At any time during the pre-bypass phase, the patient may develop life-threatening arrhythmias or severe hypotension that would necessitate proceeding quickly on bypass.
5. While the surgeon opens the mediastinum, the scrub nurse organizes and secures the extracorporeal circuit on the sterile field.	The extracorporeal circuit must be secured to the field to prevent it from falling on the floor and becoming contaminated.
6. The scrub nurse hands the distal ends of the table circuits to the perfusionist, and the circuit ends are connected to the circuits on the heart–lung machine.	It is a better aseptic technique to pass the sterile circuit ends down to the perfusionist than to have the perfusionist hand the sterile circuits up to the sterile field.
7. The perfusionist fills the arterial–venous loop with perfusate, removing all air.	This extracorporeal circuit is primed with perfusate to remove air that could cause an air embolism.
8. The perfusionist informs the scrub nurse when it is safe to divide the arterial–venous loop. The scrub nurse lets the perfusionist know when the circuits are being clamped. One line clamp is placed on both sides of the built-in connector on the arterial–venous loop. Heavy scissors are used to cut the connector out of the line. The smaller line, 3/8" in diameter, becomes the arterial circuit. The larger line, 1/2" in diameter, becomes the venous circuit. The scrub nurse has the extracorporeal circuit divided and ready to connect to the cannulas when the surgeon is ready to cannulate.	The arterial–venous circuit is divided to provide two separate circuits. The smaller circuit will become the line for arterial blood returning blood to the patient from the heart–lung machine; the larger circuit will become the venous line, directing blood from the patient to the heart–lung machine. A circuit that is clamped under pressure could cause the circuits to burst at the various connections.

Steps:	Rationale:

9. The scrub nurse prepares the cannulation stitches in the order needed. The cannulation stitches include:
   a. Aortic
   b. Atrial
   c. Antegrade cardioplegia stitch
   d. Retrograde cardioplegia stitch
   e. Vent stitch, if used
Tourniquets are placed on the suture after the stitches have been placed.
	Purse-string stitches are placed in the cannulation locations in order to secure the various perfusion cannulas during the procedure.

10. The patient is heparinized before cannulation.	Systemic anticoagulation is necessary to prevent embolization.
11. The scrub nurse hands the knife and aortic cannula to the surgeon. The distal end of the arterial cannula must be clamped, if it does not have an occlusive cap over the end. A 3/8" straight connector must be placed on the arterial table circuit if the aortic cannula does not have a connector built into the cannula.	The ascending aorta is cannulated for arterial blood return. If the arterial cannula is not capped or clamped during the insertion, blood will shoot out the end of the cannula due to the pressure in the aorta. A 3/8" connector is needed to join the extracorporeal table circuit to the aortic cannula if the cannula does not have a built-in connector.
12. After the arterial cannula is inserted into the aorta, the surgeon tightens the tourniquets. The scrub nurse has the arterial circuit ready to connect to the arterial cannula.	The tourniquets help secure the perfusion cannulas and prevent them from becoming dislodged.

Cardiac Surgery: Nursing Procedure: Institution of Cardiopulmonary Bypass

Steps:	Rationale:
13. The scrub nurse assists the surgeon in cannulating the right atrium, passing the venous cannula to the surgeon. After it is positioned, the surgeon tightens the tourniquet. The scrub nurse hands the venous circuit to the surgeon to connect to the venous cannula on the heart–lung machine for reoxygenation. The venous circuit must have a 1/2" connector on the line or a connector built in on the venous cannula to be able to connect the cannula to the circuit.	Cannulation of the right atrium sends blood to the oxygenator on the heart–lung machine for reoxygenation.
14. If the inferior and superior vena cavas are to be used instead of the right atrium for venous blood return, each cava is cannulated separately and secured with a purse-string suture and tourniquet. Umbilical cord tapes are available to go around the vena cavas. The venous circuit cannulas are connected to the venous pump circuit with a 1/2" × 1/2" × 1/2" connector.	Compression of the vena cavas with the tapes forces all the venous return into the cannulas. A 1/2" connector is needed to join the extracorporeal table to the venous cannulas.
15. The surgeon tells the perfusionist when it is time to go on bypass. Prior to initiating bypass, the perfusionist checks the ACT and the HDR.	Systemic anticoagulation is checked to ensure that the appropriate amount of heparin has been given. Perfusion is not instituted until the ACT is at least 480 seconds.
16. The scrub nurse assists the surgeon with placement of the cardioplegia cannulation stitches and cannulas.	The scrub nurse knows the routine and preference of the surgeon for cardiopulmonary bypass.

Steps:	Rationale:
17. The perfusionist fills the cardioplegia circuit. The scrub nurse ensures that the line is free of air.	Cardioplegia perfusate is pumped through the cardioplegia circuit and is ready to connect to the cardioplegia cannula. Air in the circuit could cause an air embolism.
18. The scrub nurse helps to ensure that the correct aspiration circuits are used at the appropriate times. The cell saver is used before and after cardiopulmonary bypass, and the cardiotomy suction is used after heparinization.	Blood-salvaging techniques are used to decrease the need for bank blood transfusions.
19. The perfusionist monitors the physiologic values to maintain hemostasis at regular intervals.	The laboratory values indicate to the perfusionist the metabolic, hematologic, and electrolyte status of the patient during cardiopulmonary bypass.
20. The surgeon communicates the type of myocardial protection to be instituted.	Team communication facilitates the case preparation and enables the team to plan the methods of perioperative patient care.
21. If the myocardial protection is cold intermittent cardioplegia, the circulating nurse reverses the K-thermia blanket from warm to cold. The scrub nurse turns the slush machine to the cooling mode. If warm continuous cardioplegia is utilized, a K-thermia blanket is not needed and the slush machine is maintained in the warming mode.	Myocardial protection is used to minimize ischemic damage to the myocardium, provide a motionless field, and prolong safe operating time. The type of myocardial protection is dependent on the surgeon's preference and the condition of the patient.
22. The scrub nurse maintains the integrity of the extracorporeal table circuits.	The extracorporeal circuit must remain sterile, intact, and free of kinks during cardiopulmonary bypass.

Steps:	Rationale:
23. When the surgeon tells the perfusionist to rewarm, the circulating nurse reverses the K-thermia blanket to the warming mode, and the scrub nurse reverses the slush machine to the warming mode.	The patient's systemic temperature must be returned to normal before discontinuation of cardiopulmonary bypass. Cold saline poured over a beating heart can cause the heart to fibrillate.
24. The circulating nurse is aware of the need for activation of the defibrillator. The scrub nurse has the internal defibrillating paddles available. The circulating nurse does not leave the defibrillator unattended until a regular EKG pattern has been established	Fibrillation is common when blood begins to flow again through the heart. Repeated defibrillation at higher voltages may be required to convert to a sinus rhythm.
25. After completion of the cardiac repair or revascularization, the anesthesiologist, perfusionist, and surgeon work together to wean the patient from cardiopulmonary bypass. The team anticipates the need for an intra-aortic balloon to support cardiac output if the patient cannot be weaned from cardiopulmonary bypass.	Certain hemodynamic parameters are achieved to wean a patient successfully from cardiopulmonary bypass, including an adequate cardiac rhythm, acceptable systemic pressures, normothermia, and an adequate cardiac output. An intra-aortic balloon may be inserted to augment the patient's cardiac output.
26. After the patient's hemodynamics have stabilized and the patient is weaned from cardiopulmonary bypass, protamine is administered by the anesthesiologist. The patient's hemodynamics are observed during the administration of protamine.	Protamine reverses the anticoagulant effects of the heparin. Some patients present with an anaphylactic reaction to protamine shown by a profound drop in blood pressure due to vasodilation.

Steps:	Rationale:
27. After the patient is weaned from bypass, the surgeon removes the arterial and venous cannulas. The scrub nurse assists the surgeon with the decannulation process and is prepared at all times to recannulate if it should become necessary.	If the patient's condition deteriorates, the team must be prepared to reinstitute cardiopulmonary bypass.
28. The perfusionist hemoconcentrates the blood remaining in the oxygenator and gives the processed blood to the anesthesiologist.	Blood remaining in the oxygenator is concentrated and transfused to the patient.
29. The scrub nurse maintains the integrity of the extracorporeal table circuits until the sternum has been reapproximated with wire.	The circuit remains sterile in case a sudden change in the patient's condition warrants the reinstitution of cardiopulmonary bypass.
30. After the sternum has been closed, the scrub nurse hands the extracorporeal table circuits to the perfusionist. The perfusionist removes and disposes of the pump circuits.	All pump circuits are disposed of according to hospital policy regarding contaminated trash.
31. The perfusionist cleans the heart–lung machine and gathers perfusion supplies needed for another case.	Supplies and equipment are always available should the need arise to reinstitute cardiopulmonary bypass. The pump is left clean and intact for the next case.

Standard of Care: Cardiac Surgery: Cardiopulmonary Bypass

I. Phases of Cardiopulmonary Bypass
   A. Prebypass
   B. Instituting and maintaining bypass
   C. Discontinuation of cardiopulmonary bypass
   D. Postcardiopulmonary bypass
II. Indications for Cardiopulmonary Bypass
   A. Preservation of organ viability
   B. Maintenance of near-normal hemodynamic and metabolic conditions during a temporary absence of cardiac and pulmonary function
   C. Facilitates open heart surgery on a motionless, relatively bloodless heart
      1. Used on many open-heart procedures
      2. Adult respiratory distress syndrome
      3. Used in conjunction with a left ventricular assist device to support patients awaiting heart transplantation
      4. Used as adjunct therapy for coronary arterial angioplasty and coronary stenting
III. Special Equipment
   A. Heart–lung machine
      1. Gas exchange device
         a. Oxygenator
      2. Pump
         a. Heat exchanger
         b. Arterial filter
         c. Bubble detector/level sensor
         d. Temperature monitor
   B. Extracorporeal circuits
      1. Table circuits
         a. Arterial–venous circuit
         b. Cardioplegia delivery circuit
         c. Cardiotomy aspiration circuits
            1. Vent circuit
      2. Pump circuits
   C. Perfusion cannulas
      1. Arterial
         a. Aortic
         b. Femoral artery
      2. Venous

        a. Atrial
        b. Femoral vein
        c. Inferior and superior vena cavas
   D. Stat lab equipment
      1. Blood gas analyzer
      2. Electrolyte analyzer
      3. Glucose counter
      4. ACT monitor
      5. HPT/HDR monitor
      6. Hematocrit monitor
   E. Ultrafiltration
      1. Indications
        a. Fluid overload
        b. Hyperkalemia
        c. Low hematocrit
        d. Ability to process the remaining perfusate in the extracorporeal circuit
           1. Preserves clotting factors
           2. Salvages blood left in the oxygenator reservoir
      2. Set up and primed according to manufacturer's specifications
IV. Special Considerations
   A. All staff is educated in the function of the heart–lung machine and the dynamics of cardiopulmonary bypass.
   B. All staff is familiar with the necessary equipment associated with cardiopulmonary bypass and its location.
   C. Cardiopulmonary bypass is initiated by the perfusionist under the direction and supervision of the cardiac surgeon.
   D. All team members participating in the surgical procedure are aware at all times of the patient's hemodynamic status and heparinization status.
   E. The perioperative plan of care is centered around the safe, effective, and efficient placement of the patient on cardiopulmonary bypass.
   F. Communication among all team members is essential for safety and efficiency.
   G. A perfusion protocol is written specific to the type of procedures performed, surgeon preference, and practice habits.
      1. Protocol guidelines
        a. Perfusionist availability and responsibility
        b. Heart–lung pump circuits
        c. Type of perfusate
        d. Stat lab determinations
           1. Identification of specific tests
           2. Time intervals that the labs are drawn

Standard of Care: Cardiac Surgery: Cardiopulmonary Bypass

3. Acceptable parameters of lab determinations
4. Plan of action established if values do not meet the acceptable range
   e. Calculation of flow rates
   f. Control of systemic pressure
   g. Systemic temperature regulation
   h. Documentation procedure
V. Prebypass Procedures
   A. Surgeon responsibilities
      1. Communicate to the team the type of myocardial protection
         a. Warm continuous cardioplegia delivery
         b. Cold intermittent cardioplegia delivery
         c. Systemic temperature control
      2. Communicates to the perfusionist the perfusate used to prime the extracorporeal circuits
   B. Anesthesiologist responsibilities
      1. Invasive line placement for hemodynamic monitoring
      2. Hemodynamic support, as needed, until cardiopulmonary bypass is initiated
   C. Perfusionist responsibilities
      1. Prepares the extracorporeal circuit for the heart–lung machine
      2. Gives the scrub nurse/tech the extracorporeal table circuits for the heart–lung machine
      3. Calculates the heparin dose according to the weight of the patient.
      4. Calculates the perfusion flow rates based on liters per minute per square meter of body surface area
      5. Communicates special needs to the circulating nurse
         a. Ice, if needed, for cold intermittent cardioplegia delivery
         b. Bank blood to prime the extracorporeal circuit if the patient's hematocrit is low
      6. Completes the quality assurance checks on all the stat lab equipment
      7. Performs all the prebypass lab tests
         a. Hematocrit
         b. Electrolytes
         c. Arterial and venous blood gases
         d. Activated clotting time
         e. Heparin dose response
         f. Glucose level
      8. Completes the preliminary safety checks for cardiopulmonary bypass
      9. Is constantly aware of the patient's hemodynamic status

D. Circulating nurses' responsibilities
   1. Educated in the function of the heart–lung machine and is familiar with the equipment and location of supplies needed for cardiopulmonary bypass
   2. Constantly aware of the patient's hemodynamic status
   3. Assists the scrub nurse/tech with gathering and opening the sterile perfusion supplies needed on the field
   4. Checks the patient's lab results, notifying the surgeon, anesthesiologist, and perfusionist of any abnormalities
   5. Notifies the perfusionist of the patient's height and weight
   6. Retrieves bank blood
   7. Gives heparin to the scrub nurse/tech
E. Scrub nurse/tech responsibilities
   1. Education
      a. The scrub nurse/tech is educated in the function of the heart–lung machine and the extracorporeal circuits with their specific functions.
         1. Arterial–venous loop
         2. Cardioplegia line
         3. Cardiotomy suction line
         4. Vent/cardiotomy line
      b. The scrub nurse/tech knows the diameter of each individual tubing.
         1. Facilitates the connections of the extracorporeal circuits with the various perfusion cannulas
      c. The scrub nurse/tech has a working knowledge of the cannulation process for cardiopulmonary bypass.
         1. Familiar with the different perfusion cannulas
            a. Type
               1. Arterial
               2. Venous
               3. Percutaneous arterial and venous
            b. Location
               1. Aorta
               2. Femoral artery/femoral vein
               3. Right atrium
               4. Inferior and superior vena cavas
         2. Knows the cannulation stitches
         3. Knows the surgeon's routine and preference for establishment of cardiopulmonary bypass
            a. Knows the type of myocardial protection used
               1. Prepares the slush machine with cold or warm saline

2. Gathers and opens the appropriate supplies needed for cardiopulmonary bypass
   3. Draws the correct heparin dose in a syringe for the intraoperative injection into the right atrium by the surgeon, if heparin given on the field.
   4. Organizes and secures the extracorporeal circuit to the sterile drapes while the surgeon is opening the mediastinum
   F. Hemodynamic monitoring specialist responsibilities
      1. Constantly aware of the patient's hemodynamic status
         a. The care delivered is revised, as necessary, to meet the change in the patient's hemodynamic status.
      2. Assists the anesthesiologist with invasive line placement
      3. Assists the perfusionist with the prebypass lab tests
         a. Baseline blood gas
         b. Activated clotting time
VI. Implementing and Maintaining Cardiopulmonary Bypass
   A. Surgeon responsibilities
      1. Heparin is given according to patient's body weight.
      2. Arterial and venous cannulation is accomplished.
      3. He or she communicates to the perfusionist when to start cardiopulmonary bypass
   B. Anesthesiologist responsibilities
      1. Make sure that the ventilator is turned off
      2. Communicates with the perfusionist the type of anesthetic gases or drugs to use during cardiopulmonary bypass to facilitate anesthesia
      3. May give heparin per surgeon's request
   C. Perfusionist responsibilities
      1. Assures that the extracorporeal circuits are connected appropriately and that all lines are unclamped before initiating bypass
      2. Responsible for monitoring physiologic values to maintain hemostasis at regular intervals
         a. Systemic pressure
            1. Maintains arterial blood pressure above at least 60 mm Hg for an adequate cardiac output
         b. Arterial and venous blood gases
            1. Arterial PO_2 while on bypass is maintained between 100 and 400 mm Hg.
            2. PCO_2 while on bypass is maintained between 35 and 45 mm Hg.
            3. Arterial pH is maintained above 7.30 with normal PCO_2.
         c. Hematocrit
            1. Maintained above 20%

d. Electrolytes
      1. Potassium
      2. Sodium
      3. Glucose
   e. Activated clotting time
      1. Perfusion is not instituted until the ACT is at least 480 seconds
   f. Heparin/protamine titration
      1. HPT must be at least 3.0 mg/kg.
   g. Monitors the urine output
D. Circulating nurse responsibilities
   1. Checks the bank blood with the perfusionist as needed
   2. Opens the necessary supplies for the scrub nurse/tech
   3. Assists the perfusionist, as needed, communication with the scrub nurse/tech, and any additional supplies that might be needed
   4. Assists with systemic temperature control
      a. The K-thermia blanket is reversed from warm to cold if using cold myocardial protection techniques
   5. The internal paddles are connected to the defibrillator.
E. Scrub nurse/tech responsibilities
   1. Keeps in constant, direct communication with the perfusionist
   2. The extracorporeal table circuit is ready when the surgeon starts to cannulate.
      a. The arterial–venous circuit is divided after the line has been filled with perfusate and the perfusionist gives the consent to divide.
   3. Assists the surgeon with the cannulation process
      a. Passes the correct cannulation stitches in the order used
      b. Passes the appropriate cannulas
      c. Has the appropriate extracorporeal circuits ready to connect to the cannulas
   4. Maintains the integrity of the extracorporeal table circuit
      a. Prevents kinks in the circuits
      b. Is aware, at all times, of the location and the function of all the various circuits
   5. Facilitates the method of myocardial protection
      a. If cold intermittent cardioplegia is used.
         1. Slush or cold saline is available.
         2. Warm saline is available as the patient is rewarmed.
         3. Assures that the internal paddles are available
      b. If warm continuous cardioplegia is used
         1. Warm saline is available throughout the duration of the procedure.

6. Communicates the progression of the case to the perfusionist
7. Facilitates the use of the appropriate aspiration circuits during cardiopulmonary bypass
   a. Cardiotomy suction is used for blood lost after systemic heparinization and during cardiopulmonary bypass.
   b. The cell saver suction is used to remove slush or irrigating fluids during cardiopulmonary bypass.
F. Hemodynamic monitoring specialist
   1. Assists the perfusionist and circulating nurse as needed
VII. Discontinuation of Cardiopulmonary Bypass
   A. Parameters for discontinuation of cardiopulmonary bypass
      1. Completion of the cardiac repair or revascularization procedure
      2. Adequate cardiac output
      3. Acceptable systemic arterial blood pressure
      4. Adequate filling pressures
         a. Pulmonary artery diastolic pressures
         b. CVP
      5. Acceptable cardiac rhythm
      6. Acceptable electrolyte balance
      7. Core temperature within normal limits
   B. Surgeon responsibilities
      1. Air is removed from the heart after the repair or revascularization process is completed.
      2. Hemostasis is accomplished.
      3. The patient is rewarmed.
      4. The surgeon directs the perfusionist to slowly wean the patient from cardiopulmonary bypass.
      5. After patient is stabilized and off bypass, protamine is started.
      6. Arterial and venous cannulas are removed and purse-string sutures around the insertion sites are tied.
   C. Anesthesiologist responsibilities
      1. Ventilates the patient
      2. Returns to the prebypass mode, with stabilization of the patient's hemodynamics
      3. Regulates the appropriate fluid volume
      4. Delivers the appropriate protamine dose
   D. Perfusionist responsibilities
      1. All lab values are evaluated.
         a. Serum potassium within normal limits.
         b. Acid–base status is normal.
         c. Core temperature is above 35° centigrade.
         d. Cardiac rhythm is stable.

            e. Pulmonary filling pressures are within normal limits.
                1. Pulmonary artery pressure is maintained at, or near, 15–20 mm Hg.
            f. Arterial pressure is acceptable.
        2. Slowly weans the patient off of cardiopulmonary bypass under the direction of the surgeon
            a. Flow rates are decreased slowly, evaluating the patient's response.
        3. The perfusionist transfers the oxygenator volume in the direction of the patient to maintain mean pulmonary artery pressures at or near 15–20 mm Hg unless advised otherwise by the surgeon.
        4. The oxygenator reservoir is not depleted beyond the level of fluid that would permit reinstitution of bypass until specific and confirmed approval of the surgeon has been given.
        5. Unused volume remaining in the oxygenator reservoir is passed through a hemofilter, infused into a transfer pack, and delivered to the anesthesiologist.
        6. The cardiotomy suction is turned off after 50% of the protamine has been given.
        7. The pump and oxygenator are maintained in working order until the patient is stable and the sternal wires are placed.
    E. Circulating nurse responsibilities
        1. Assists the perfusionist and scrub nurse/tech as needed
        2. Is constantly aware of the patient's hemodynamic status
    F. Scrub nurse/tech responsibilities
        1. Assists the surgeon with the decannulation process
        2. Extra cannulation sutures are available as needed
        3. Is constantly aware of the patient's hemodynamic status
            a. Is ready, at all times, to reinstitute cardiopulmonary bypass, if the need arises
            b. Maintains the integrity of the extracorporeal table circuits until the sternum has been reapproximated with wire
        4. Passes the extracorporeal table circuits to the perfusionist after the sternal wires have been positioned and the chest reapproximated
    G. Hemodynamic monitoring specialist responsibilities
        1. Blood in the cell saver is spun and washed in the cell saver and returned in a transfusion bag to the anesthesiologist.
        2. Assists the anesthesiologist, perfusionist, and circulating nurse, as needed
VIII. Postbypass
    A. Surgeon responsibilities
        1. Wound closure

            2. Hemostasis
        B. Anesthesiologist responsibilities
            1. Monitors the hemodynamic status
            2. Completes the anesthesia record
            3. Pain management
        C. Perfusionist responsibilities
            1. Assists with the postbypass lab determinations
                a. Hematocrit
                b. Blood gases
                c. Electrolytes
                d. HPT
                e. Glucose
            2. Disconnects the extracorporeal circuits on the heart–lung machine and disposes of them according to hospital policy
            3. Completes the perfusion record
            4. Cleans the heart–lung machine
            5. Remains in the surgery department until the patient has been transferred to the intensive care unit
            6. Retrieves supplies needed for the next case
        D. Circulating nurse
            1. Assists the team in the hemodynamic stability of the patient
        E. Scrub nurse/tech responsibilities
            1. Assists the team with maintaining hemostasis
        F. Hemodynamic monitoring specialist responsibilities
            1. Assists the team with maintaining the hemodynamic stability of the patient
IX. Inability to Wean the Patient from Cardiopulmonary Bypass
        A. Maintenance of cardiopulmonary bypass for circulatory support until other definitive measures can be instituted
        B. Guidelines to definitive action
            1. Bleeding is controlled.
            2. Temporary pacing wires are positioned to maintain an adequate rhythm.
            3. Cardiac supportive drug therapy is instituted.
            4. An intra-aortic balloon may be used.
            5. An LVAD/RVAD may be used.
        C. Communication with the intensive care unit
X. Documentation of Cardiopulmonary Bypass
        A. Responsibility of the perfusionist
        B. Guidelines to specific documentation required
            1. Patient's name, age, sex, weight, height, and body surface area
            2. Date of procedure

3. Patient's medical record number
4. Diagnosis
5. Procedure performed
6. Patient allergies
7. The names of the surgeon, cardiologist, perfusionist, and anesthesiologist
8. Manufacturer and serial number of the oxygenator
9. Manufacturer and lot number of the extracorporeal circuits
10. Manufacturer of the arterial filter
11. Heparin dose and time given
12. Pump prime
13. Safety checklist
14. Fluid intake
    a. Bank blood given by the anesthesiologist
    b. Prebypass fluid
    c. Total pump prime
    d. Fluid on cardiopulmonary bypass
    e. Colloid on cardiopulmonary bypass
    f. Blood on cardiopulmonary bypass
    g. Crystalloid
    h. Total intake
15. Fluid loss
    a. Estimated blood loss
    b. Urine output prebypass
    c. Urine output during cardiopulmonary bypass
    d. Ultrafiltrate
    e. Total fluid loss
    f. Net gain or loss
16. Cardioplegia perfusate
17. Type of cardioplegia delivery
18. Time cardioplegia is delivered
19. Amount of cardioplegia delivered
20. Method of venting
21. Times cardiopulmonary bypass is instituted and discontinued
    a. Patient's response before and after bypass
22. Total cross-clamp time
23. Medications used and time used
24. Cardiopulmonary flow rates
25. Lab determinations
    a. Names of specific tests
    b. Time drawn
    c. Results

    d. Definitive action taken
  26. Hemodynamic parameters
    a. Mean arterial pressure
    b. CVP pressures
    c. Core temperatures
  27. Amount and type of anesthetic gas delivered
  28. Additional comments
XI. Maintenance of the Heart–Lung Machine
  A. As soon as a problem arises
  B. Routine maintenance completed according to the manufacturer's recommendations
XII. Clinical Indicators for Evaluation
  A. Staff education pertaining to cardiopulmonary bypass
    1. Individual team roles
    2. Effective communication between team members
    3. An emergency plan of care established for quick implementation of bypass
    4. Location of perfusion supplies
  B. Availability of pertinent perfusion supplies
  C. Time needed to prepare for cardiopulmonary bypass
  D. Time needed to implement cardiopulmonary bypass
  E. Patient's expected response to cardiopulmonary bypass
  F. Patient's actual response to cardiopulmonary bypass
  G. Pertinent documentation of perfusion
  H. Maintenance of the heart–lung machine

THE EXTRACORPOREAL CIRCUT

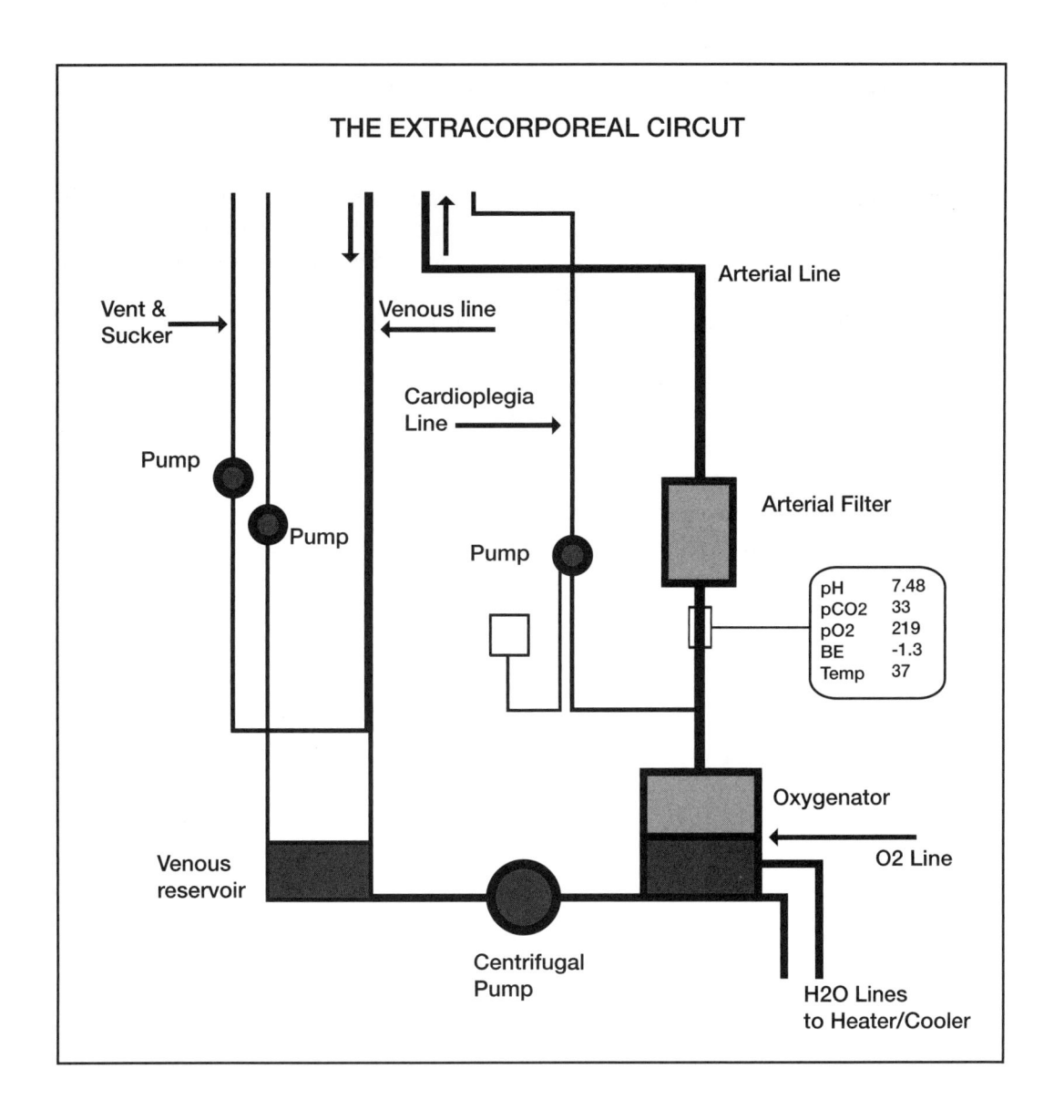

- Vent & Sucker
- Venous line
- Arterial Line
- Pump
- Pump
- Cardioplegia Line
- Pump
- Arterial Filter

pH	7.48
pCO2	33
pO2	219
BE	-1.3
Temp	37

- Venous reservoir
- Oxygenator
- O2 Line
- Centrifugal Pump
- H2O Lines to Heater/Cooler

Standard of Care: Cardiac Surgery: Cardiopulmonary Bypass

Cardiac Surgery: Policy: Myocardial Protection

Cardiac surgery's policy is that the intraoperative myocardial protection technique be determined by the physician. The techniques used are communicated to the cardiac team to enable them to plan the methods with which to provide the care to achieve the optimal patient response.

Planning includes but is not limited to the following:

1. Organization of special supplies and equipment
2. Maintenance of requested systemic temperatures
3. Correct utilization of the slush machine and K-thermia unit at the appropriate time
4. Methods aimed at decreasing the metabolic needs of the patient
5. Methods aimed at ensuring that the oxygen supply meets the oxygen demands of the patient

Cardiac Surgery: Nursing Procedure: Myocardial Protection Utilizing Cold Intermittent Cardioplegia

Quality Outcome: Myocardial energy resources are preserved by manually arresting the heart during cardiopulmonary bypass, lowering the systemic temperature, and cooling the heart. This enables the surgeon to work in a motionless, bloodless field, allowing direct vision of the heart.

Performed by: Surgeon, perfusionist, circulating nurse, and scrub nurse

General Statement: The cardiac team is prepared to meet the following criteria:

1. Supplies and equipment are available.
2. A perioperative plan of care is devised for cardioplegia delivery, hypothermia, and reversing the hypothermic conditions at the appropriate time.

Equipment: Perfusate, blood, or crystalloid cardioplegia, composition determined by the physician; extracorporeal circuit for the cardioplegia delivery; antegrade catheter; retrograde catheter; appropriate sutures and tourniquets; Frazier suction tip; slush machine with the capability to heat and cool; defibrillator; saline (2 to 3 liters); K-thermia unit and corresponding blanket; temperature monitors that may include but are not limited to (a) esophageal, (b) bladder, and (c) rectal; and myocardial temporary pacing wires.

Steps:

1. The surgeon communicates the type of myocardial protection technique to the cardiac team perioperatively.
   Details include but are not limited to
   a. Hypothermia or normothermia
   b. Composition of the cardioplegia
   c. Site of cardioplegia delivery
      1. Antegrade
      2. Retrograde
      3. Antegrade and retrograde
      4. Vein grafts
      5. Intracoronary

Rationale:

Team communication facilitates the initial case preparation and enables the team to plan the methods of perioperative patient care.

Steps:	Rationale:
2. The scrub nurse gathers and opens, on the sterile field, the cardioplegia cannula or cannulas, slush drape, extracorporeal cardioplegia delivery circuit for use on the surgical field, sutures, and tourniquets.	The scrub nurse's responsibility is to ensure that all lines, cannulas, and sutures for cannulation are assembled.
3. The scrub nurse drapes the slush machine.	The drape provides a sterile barrier for the sterile saline.
4. The circulating nurse pours 2 to 3 liters of cold saline into the basin of the slush machine. The cooling mode is turned to the "on" position.	The saline must be precooled to decrease the amount of time needed to prepare slush.
5. The circulating nurse places the K-thermia blanket under the sheet of the surgical table preoperatively. The blanket is connected to the K-thermia unit. The unit is checked to ensure the correct temperature. Initially, the blanket may be turned to the warming mode for patient comfort during the invasive line placement.	The blanket must be positioned on the surgical table before transfer of the patient from the gurney to the surgical table if the blanket is to be positioned underneath the patient. Blankets that are placed around the periphery of the patient are placed before the surgical prep. The blanket must be padded to prevent the possibility of burns. Shivering increases the metabolic demands of the patient, requiring a higher oxygen consumption.
6. After induction of the patient, the circulating nurse positions the appropriate temperature monitor. This may consist of but is not limited to a. Rectal or bladder All bony prominences are padded.	The temperature probes will monitor systemic temperatures intraoperatively. Padding reduces pressure injuries.

Steps:	Rationale:
7. The perfusionist prepares the cardioplegia circuit for the heart–lung machine. A bucket of ice is available.	The perfusionist is responsible for the assembly of the circuits needed for cardiopulmonary bypass. The ice is added to the heater–cooler on the heart–lung machine and around the cardioplegia circuit to facilitate systemic cooling.
8. While the sternotomy is being made, the scrub nurse secures the pump tubing and cardioplegia delivery circuit to the surgical drapes, determining the length of the circuits needed on the surgical field, and handing the ends that need to be connected to the heart–lung machine to the perfusionist.	To maintain sterility, the extracorporeal circuit is passed down from the surgical field to the heart–lung machine.
9. The scrub nurse assists the surgeon and the assistant with the cardioplegia cannulation stitches, tourniquets, and cannulation of the cardioplegia catheter(s). The cardioplegia delivery circuit is connected to the cardioplegia catheters. A myocardial temperature probe may be placed on the myocardium.	The scrub nurse knows the surgeon's routine and preferences for cannulation. The stitches and tourniquets provide stabilization of the cardioplegia catheters to prevent accidental dislodgement. The temperature probe monitors myocardial temperature.
10. The cardioplegia line is filled with perfusate by the perfusionist and the scrub nurse after the initiation of cardiopulmonary bypass. The scrub nurse checks to ensure that all air bubbles are removed from the cardioplegia line before handing the line to the surgeon to connect to the appropriate cardioplegia cannula/cannulas.	The cardioplegia solution is cooled and maintained at a predetermined temperature for optimum myocardial protection.

Steps:	Rationale:
11. The scrub nurse connects the cardiotomy suction tip to an aspiration line.	Air in the delivery system could cause air embolism.
12. The aortic cross clamp is placed across the aorta by the surgeon. The surgeon requests that the cardioplegia be started, and the patient is cooled. Cardioplegia is infused every 15 to 20 minutes to maintain cardiac arrest.	Cold cardioplegic arrest is accomplished by infusing the coronary arteries with a cold, high-potassium concentration and various buffering agents to counteract ischemic acidosis. The aorta is occluded to block systemic circulation and facilitates the cardioplegia delivery to the myocardium.
13. The K-thermia blanket is reversed to the cooling mode.	Cold cardioplegia in conjunction with systemic hypothermia reduces energy requirements of the myocardium.
14. Slush or cold saline is poured over the myocardium.	Local hypothermia is used to cool the myocardium further.
15. After the surgical repair is completed, the surgeon will alert the perfusionist to "rewarm." The blood circulating in the heart–lung machine is warmed, and the cardioplegia is discontinued. The circulating nurse turns the K-thermia blanket to the warming mode. The scrub nurse turns the warming mode on the slush machine. The EKG is monitored for a return heartbeat or fibrillation.	The patient's systemic temperature is returned to normal, and the cardioplegia solution is flushed out of the collateral circulation. The heart may fibrillate or convert spontaneously.
16. The circulating nurse is ready to charge the defibrillator if necessary.	Internal paddles are available to treat ventricular fibrillation with countershock.
17. All irrigation used is warm.	Normothermic conditions are maintained. Cold irrigation on a beating heart may cause ventricular fibrillation.

Steps:	Rationale:
18. The scrub nurse has temporary pacing wires available.	Pacing may be necessary to treat dysrhythmias.
19. After discontinuation of cardiopulmonary bypass and the patient is hemodynamically stable, the cardioplegia circuit on the field is passed to the perfusionist.	Hemoconcentration of the blood remaining in the oxygenator reservoir is accomplished using the cardioplegia delivery circuit.

Cardiac Surgery: Nursing Procedure: Myocardial Protection Using Warm Continuous Cardioplegia

Quality Outcome: Cardiac arrest is induced during cardiopulmonary bypass using continuous, warm, aerobic perfusion, maximizing oxygen supply, minimizing demand, and providing a motionless field in which to operate.

Performed by: Surgeon, perfusionist, circulating nurse, and scrub nurse

General Statement: The cardiac team has the supplies, equipment, and a plan of care necessary to deliver continuous, warm, aerobic cardioplegia during the cardiac surgical procedure.

Equipment: Perfusate, blood cardioplegia, composition determined by the physician; extracorporeal circuit for cardioplegia delivery, antegrade cardioplegia catheter, retrograde cardioplegia catheter, pressure line and transducer; appropriate sutures and tourniquets, Frazier suction tip, slush machine with the capability to heat and cool; defibrillator; and saline, 2 to 3 liters

Steps:	Rationale:

1. The surgeon communicates the type of myocardial protection technique to the cardiac team preoperatively. Details include but are not limited to
  a. Normothermia or hypothermia
  b. Composition of the cardioplegia
  c. Site of the cardioplegia delivery
    1. Antegrade
    2. Retrograde
    3. Antegrade and retrograde
    4. Vein grafts
    5. Intracoronary
	Team communication facilitates the initial case preparation and enables the team to plan the methods of perioperative patient care.

2. The scrub nurse gathers and opens, on the sterile field, the cardioplegia cannula or cannulas, slush drape, the extracorporeal cardioplegia delivery circuit for use on the surgical field, sutures, and tourniquets.	It is the scrub nurse's responsibility to ensure that all lines, cannulas, and sutures for cannulation are assembled.

Steps:	Rationale:
3. The scrub nurse drapes the slush machine.	The drape provides a sterile barrier for the sterile saline.
4. The circulating nurse pours 2 to 3 liters of room-temperature saline into the basin of the slush machine. The warming mode is not turned on until the basin on the slush machine is filled with saline.	Saline is used for irrigation. Without liquid in the bottom of the slush machine, the drape will melt against the warm metal.
5. The perfusionist prepares the cardioplegia delivery circuit for the heart–lung machine.	The perfusionist is responsible for the assembly of the circuits needed for cardiopulmonary bypass.
6. While the sternotomy is being made, the scrub nurse secures the pump tubing and cardioplegia delivery circuit to the surgical drapes, determining the length of the circuits needed on the surgical field, and handing the ends that need to be connected to the heart–lung machine to the perfusionist.	To maintain sterility, the extracorporeal circuit is passed down from the surgical field to the heart–lung machine.
7. The scrub nurse assists the surgeon and assistant with the cardioplegia cannulation stitches, tourniquets, and cannulation of the cardioplegia catheter(s). The cardioplegia delivery circuit is connected to the cardioplegia catheters. A pressure line is connected to a port on the retrograde catheter to measure the pressure under which the cardioplegia is delivered.	The scrub nurse knows the surgeon's routine and preferences for cannulation. The stitches and tourniquets provide stabilization of the cardioplegia catheters to prevent accidental dislodgement. Between 30 and 60 millimeters of pressure are needed to deliver the cardioplegia to the coronary arteries through the retrograde catheter.

Nursing Procedure: Myocardial Protection Using Warm Continuous Cardioplegia

Steps:	Rationale:
8. The cardioplegia line is filled with perfusate by the perfusionist and the scrub nurse after the initiation of cardiopulmonary bypass. The scrub nurse checks to ensure that all air bubbles are removed from the cardioplegia line before handing the line to the surgeon to connect to the appropriate cardioplegia cannulas.	Blood collected in the heart–lung oxygenator/reservoir during bypass is a necessary component for aerobic cardioplegia delivery. Utilization of bank blood is not necessary. Air in the delivery system could cause air embolism.
9. The aortic cross clamp is placed across the aorta by the surgeon. The cardioplegia delivery is begun and is continuous throughout the duration of cardiopulmonary bypass.	The aorta is occluded to block systemic circulation and facilitates the cardioplegia delivery to the myocardium.
10. The scrub nurse connects the Frazier suction tip to the aspiration or filtered air delivery system.	The immediate surgical field is kept dry either by aspiration or by blowing filtered CO_2 to facilitate the surgeon's field of vision during the repair or revascularization procedure.
11. All irrigation used is warm. Laps are moistened with warm saline, if needed.	All attempts are made to maintain the patient at normal body temperature.
12. The internal paddles are connected to the defibrillator and ready for use.	Ventricular fibrillation may occur as the high potassium level of the cardioplegia solution diminishes and the heart attempts to eject.
13. After discontinuation of cardiopulmonary bypass and the patient is hemodynamically stable, the cardioplegia circuit on the field is passed to the perfusionist.	Hemoconcentration of the blood is performed with the remaining volume in the oxygenated reservoir.

Standard of Care: Cardiac Surgery: Myocardial Protection

I. Goals of Myocardial Protection
   A. Minimize ischemic damage to the myocardium
   B. Provide a motionless field
   C. Prolong safe operating time
II. Phases of Myocardial Protection
   A. Preoperative interventions
      1. Pharmacologic management
      2. PTCA
      3. Thrombolytic therapy
   B. Intraoperative interventions
      1. Adequate oxygen supply, meeting the demands
      2. Hemodynamic stability
      3. Adequate perfusion of cardioplegia solution and systemic temperature monitoring
   C. Postoperative interventions
      1. Maintaining adequate cardiac outputs
      2. Maintaining adequate oxygenation
III. Types of Myocardial Protection
   A. Chemical perfusate
      1. Optimize the ratio of energy supply to consumption
      2. Optimize the capacity of the heart to use oxygen
         a. Aerobic metabolism
         b. Anaerobic metabolism
   B. Systemic temperature control
   C. Topical temperature control
   D. Oxygen delivery
   E. Hemodynamic stability
IV. Determination of Myocardial Protection Techniques
   A. Physical condition of the patient
   B. Physician's preference
   C. Type of cardiac procedure
   D. Length of procedure
V. Chemical Perfusate Components
   A. Chemical
      1. Potassium
         a. High concentration
         b. Low concentration
   B. Composition

    1. Crystalloid
    2. Blood
   C. Temperature
    1. Warm
    2. Cold
   D. Technique in which it is delivered
    1. Continuous
    2. Intermittent
    3. The pressure at which it is delivered
   E. Duration of time the perfusate is delivered
   F. Site of delivery
    1. Antegrade
    2. Retrograde
    3. Intracoronary
    4. Vein graft
VI. Systemic Temperature Control
   A. Hypothermic
   B. Normothermic
VII. Local Temperature Control
   A. Topical slush
   B. Cold saline
   C. Warm saline
   D. K-thermia machine with blanket
VIII. Intraoperative Considerations
   A. Cardioplegia delivery system
    1. Extracorporeal circuit
    2. Antegrade perfusion catheter
    3. Retrograde perfusion catheter
    4. Intracoronary perfusion catheter
   B. Slush machine to heat or cool saline
   C. Temperature probes may be used
    1. Esophageal temperature probe
    2. Rectal or bladder temperature probe
    3. Extracorporeal circuit temperature monitor
    4. Myocardial temperature probe
   D. K-thermia machine may be used to heat or cool
   E. Devices used to clear surgical site during cardioplegia delivery
    1. Frazier suction tip
     a. Connected to suction to aspirate at the surgical site
     b. Connected to filtered air to blow the field dry
    2. Left pulmonary vein vent
    3. Antegrade vent line

      F. The internal defibrillator paddles are connected to the defibrillator and ready for use should the need arise.
      G. Temporary pacing wires and a pulse generator are available.
IX. Clinical Indicators for Evaluation
      A. Patient's response to myocardial protection
      B. Patient outcomes
      C. Staff education
          1. Warm cardioplegia
          2. Cold cardioplegia

Off-Pump Procedures

Myocardial revascularization accomplished through the CABG procedure may be attempted and performed on a beating heart without the use of the heart–lung machine.

Off-pump procedures are determined by the patient's physical condition at the time of surgery, the coronary arteries involved and their location on the heart, and the physician's diagnosis. Scheduling of these procedures may be complex and require last-minute determinations based on the patient's immediate needs. Patients may be scheduled as off-pump procedures, may start out as off-pump cases and turn into the need for CPB, or may be a combination of off-pump and CPB procedures.

The sequence of events for off-pump procedures is carried out as standard CABG with use of the heart–lung machine but entails close monitoring of the patient's hemodynamic status at all times by the entire healthcare team and the ability to place the patient on cardiopulmonary bypass emergently, as the need arises.

The anesthesiologist and perfusionist remain in the surgical suite at all times.

The heart–lung machine is primed and the perfusionist is ready to initiate cardiopulmonary bypass if the patient becomes hemodynamically unstable. The scrub nurse at the field has the sutures available and maintains the ability to facilitate cannulation needed for cardiopulmonary bypass throughout the procedure.

Preoperatively, the patient is assessed the same as any cardiac surgical patient prior to transport to surgery. The baseline lab values are critical to analyze whether the patient may be a candidate for off-pump procedures. Since oxygen delivery is already compromised through the obstructed coronary artery, it is essential that the preoperative patient have a good hematocrit and hemoglobin to maintain oxygenation with an adequate blood pressure to support the blood flow. The patient's acid–base balance and electrolyte status must be stabilized to maintain normal rhythm throughout the procedure.

Intraoperatively, the patient is connected to hemodynamic monitoring devices and invasive lines placed for any cardiac surgical procedure. The positioning of the patient is supine with arms tucked at the patient's sides bilaterally as indicated for CABG procedure.

Off-pump procedures do require additional safety procedures in place prior to induction. Defibrillating pads are placed on the patient prior to induction in case immediate defibrillation is indicated at any time throughout the procedure.

Normal thermia is maintained by utilization of a heating blanket placed under the patient or around the periphery of the patient.

If the patient's hematocrit and hemoglobin are below normal limits, blood transfusion may be indicated prior to induction.

Cardiosupportive drugs may be prepared and ready to infuse to support the patient's rhythm and blood pressure throughout the procedure.

To perform surgery on a beating heart, a vacuum-assisted positioning device is placed on the heart surrounding the coronary artery to be bypassed. This vacuum device holds the heart in place and limits the mobility of the heart's pumping action while the surgeon sutures the vein or artery in place. A misting and blowing device connected to saline and carbon dioxide is utilized intraoperatively on the field to facilitate visualization during the suturing process.

The saline mist keeps the myocardium moist, and the carbon dioxide gas flow, which dissipates without danger of air embolism to the open coronary artery, maintains a dry field. The coronary arteries located on the back of the heart offer a challenge when using the off-pump vacuum-assisted retractor due to the need to place the heart on end while suturing. Communication between the surgeon and anesthesiologist is critical to maintain the patient's hemodynamic status while the positioning of the off-pump retractor and suturing is completed. Many times, the anesthesiologist utilizes the cardiosupportive drugs to maintain a hyperdynamic status to maintain adequate circulation and oxygenation to all parts of the patient's body during times that the heart may be inverted upward.

Blood flow to the individual coronary arteries may be maintained during the suturing procedure with the use of coronary shunts placed temporarily inside the coronary artery. These shunts present in different sizes and require the scrub and circulating nurse to maintain a shunt count. Sutures may also be placed around the coronary artery as a tourniquet to facilitate visualization.

The patient's family and the intensive care unit are kept updated as to the surgical progression.

The intraoperative documentation reflects the off-pump summary of the procedure along with the supportive protocol required.

Upon completion of the surgical procedure, the patient may or may not be extubated and transported to the intensive care unit as with a standard CABG procedure.

Aorta-Coronary Artery Bypass: CABG

Coronary artery disease with intractable angina pectoris is an indication for revascularization of the myocardium.

Unstable angina, acute myocardial infarction, and postinfarction cardiogenic shock are other conditions in which an operation could be beneficial.

Signs of an ischemic heart can be seen on the EKG. Depending on the location of the ischemia, the S-T segments may be elevated or depressed. If the conduction area is involved, arrhythmias may be present. The degree and severity of the infarction may cause poor ventricular function, low cardiac output, and cardiogenic shock.

The myocardium affected by the obstructed coronary arteries is revascularized by bypassing the obstruction with the use of autogenous saphenous veins, radial arteries, or, when possible, an internal mammary artery, as conduits.

This procedure may involve two separate sterile setups to prevent cross-contamination from the legs to the chest and uses two separate scrub nurses. Radial artery harvesting may also utilize an additional setup or may be shared.

Patients scheduled for coronary bypass grafting are shaved from the neck to toes bilaterally. The surgical prep requires two circulating nurses, one on each side of the patient. The chest is scrubbed first, working down toward the extremities, leaving the feet for last. The arms, if used for radial artery harvesting, may be prepped at this time as well. The patient is draped, leaving the legs exposed.

The assistant surgeon, with the help of the second circulator, who scrubs after the prep, harvests and prepares the vein/artery grafts. The amount and length of the veins harvested are dependent on the number of the arteries to be bypassed, the location on the heart, and the size of the heart. The vein must have an external diameter of at least 3.5 mm. Veins of poor quality are avoided. Veins with small lumens have the propensity to clot, reducing the blood flow to the obstructed area. When the veins and/or radial artery are removed, they are flushed and distended with a heparinized solution. All of the branches of the saphenous vein and radial artery are tied and ligated. Any constricting adventitial bands are removed. Each vein is tested for leaks. The veins and/or radial artery are stored in a bowl containing heparinized solution until needed. Careful handling and storage of the veins and arteries is important to minimize damage to the intimal layer, deposition of platelets and leukocytes on the intima, contraction damage to the smooth muscle mechanisms, and disruption of the extracellular matrix.

While the conduits are being harvested, the primary surgeon, with the assistance of the first scrub nurse, opens the chest and prepares the patient for cardiopulmonary bypass or an off-pump procedure. Once on bypass, if used, the heart is chemically arrested and perfused with vital nutrients; the core body temperature is lowered to minimize metabolism and oxygen needs, and the obstructed coronary arteries are identified. The distal end of the vein graft is sewn to the coronary artery using an end-to-side anastomosis. The proximal end of the vein is then distended, measured for the appropriate length, and sewn to the aorta, delivering oxygenated blood to the ischemic myocardium.

After hemostasis is accomplished and the hemodynamics are stabilized, the patient is weaned from cardiopulmonary bypass.

If the procedure is completed off pump, the patient remains normalthermic and the heart continues to beat throughout the procedure. The surgeon uses an off-pump retractor positioned over the affected coronary artery to provide stabilization of the heart and facilitate the anastomosis process. Small intracoronary shunts are used to provide blood flow through the artery being bypassed. The aorta is partially occluded to enable the surgeon to anastamose the conduit(s) to the aorta, which is the major blood supply for the obstructed coronary artery.

The leg and arm wounds are irrigated with an antibiotic solution. Drains are placed as needed, and the harvesting sites are closed as soon as possible and wrapped with Kerlix rolls and Ace bandages. The Ace bandages decrease peripheral edema in the extremities and help prevent venous stasis and thrombus formation. After the leg and/or arm wounds are closed, the legs are covered with a sterile drape sheet, and the instruments used on the legs are rolled to the periphery of the room. The setup is not contaminated until the patient is weaned from cardiopulmonary bypass and is hemodynamically stable, in the event more conduits are needed.

Standard of Care: Cardiac Surgery: Aorta–Coronary Bypass Surgery

I. Indications for Aorta–Coronary Artery Bypass (CABG)
   A. CAD
   B. Unstable angina unresponsive to medical therapy
   C. Acute myocardial infarction
   D. Postinfarction cardiogenic shock
II. Sign of an Ischemic Myocardium
   A. EKG changes
      1. ST segment changes
         a. Elevated
         b. Depressed
   B. Arrhythmias
   C. Poor ventricular failure
   D. Low cardiac output
   E. Cardiogenic shock
III. Revascularization of the Myocardium
   A. Location of the coronary obstruction
   B. Coronary graft conduits
      1. Saphenous vein grafts
         a. Greater saphenous
         b. Lesser saphenous
      2. Internal mammary artery
         a. Left
         b. Right
      3. Radial artery
         a. Left
         b. Right
      4. Gastric-epiploic artery
      5. Cephalic veins
      6. Synthetic grafts
      7. Donor vein
IV. Preoperative Preparation of the Patient
   A. Medical and physical assessment
   B. Preoperative diagnostic testing
   C. Preoperative lab determinations
   D. Preoperative education
   E. Signed surgical consents
   F. CABG surgical shave prep
   G. Nursing assessment

        H. Vital signs
        I. NPO
V. Preoperative Room Preparation
    A. Circulating nurse
        1. Assists the scrub nurse/tech to gather and open the appropriate supplies needed for the case
            a. The basic heart pan of instruments
            b. Conduit-harvesting instruments
        2. All equipment needed is accounted for and functioning.
        3. Counts needles, sponges, and instruments with the scrub nurse
        4. Pours saline into the slush machine
        5. The scrub nurse/tech is given the heparin and any other necessary medication for use on the sterile field.
        6. Assists the hemodynamic monitoring specialist with fluid line and cardiac supportive drug preparation
        7. Sends for the blood from the blood bank
        8. Positions the patient on the surgical table
        9. Placement of noninvasive monitoring equipment
        10. Places chest films on the x-ray view box
    B. Scrub nurse/tech
        1. Prepares the instrumentation and sutures needed for the surgical procedure
            a. Organizes a mayo stand with equipment needed for the conduit harvesting
            b. Organizes a mayo stand with instrumentation needed for the median sternotomy
        2. Completes the required sponge, needle, and instrument counts
    C. Hemodynamic monitoring specialist
        1. Prepares the invasive lines needed by the anesthesiologist
        2. Gathers the appropriate drugs needed by the anesthesiologist for the case
        3. Assists the anesthesiologist with the invasive line placement and induction of the patient
    D. Perfusionist
        1. Prepares the heart–lung machine
        2. Runs the quality assurance checks on the stat lab equipment
        3. Completes the preoperative lab determinations needed before cardiopulmonary bypass
        4. Calculates the required heparin dose
        5. Supports the team during off-pump procedures
VI. CABG Positioning
    A. Supine

1. Ulnar pads are placed around the elbows and ankles.
2. Arms are tucked at the sides after placement of invasive monitoring lines.
3. Legs are exposed for saphenous vein harvesting.
4. Arms may be exposed for radial artery harvesting.
5. Padded roll is placed under the shoulders.
6. A birdcage or mayo stand is placed over the patient's head.
7. A leg holder is positioned at the foot of the bed to facilitate the circumferential leg prep.
8. The legs are frogged after completion of the surgical prep with towels placed under the knees.
9. If an IMA is to be harvested, the table holder is positioned on the bed at the appropriate level.
10. The dispersive electrode pads are applied to the flank and buttock.

VII. Noninvasive and Invasive Physiologic Monitoring
 A. Noninvasive equipment
  1. BP cuff
  2. Pulse oximeter
  3. EKG electrodes
 B. Invasive equipment
  1. Arterial line
  2. Swan-Ganz line
  3. Peripheral IV
  4. Foley catheter

VIII. CABG Surgical Prep
 A. Performed by two circulating nurses, one on each side of the patient
  1. The prep starts at the chest, working down toward the extremities, leaving the feet/arms for last.
  2. The leg(s) and/or arm(s) are prepped circumferentially.

IX. Surgical Draping
 A. The anterior chest, abdomen, and legs are exposed.
  1. The sternal incision site is isolated with towels.
  2. A towel is placed over the perineum.
  3. A plastic "U" drape and a paper drape are placed under the legs.
  4. An extra-large plastic Ioban incise drape is applied over the towels, extending from the sternal notch to the femoral area.
  5. A CV fenestrated drape is positioned, with the sides of the drapes run along the edge of the surgical table.
  6. Stockinettes are placed over the toes and ankles.
  7. If harvesting the radial artery, the arm is placed on an armboard, sterile towel wrapped around the upper arm, and an extremity drape is used. The arm is positioned with palm side up.

X. Intraoperative Procedure
   A. The scrub nurse/tech moves the mayo stands into place.
      1. The instruments for the vein-harvesting procedure are positioned at the foot of the bed. The instruments for the radial artery harvesting are positioned near the arm being used.
         a. The second circulator becomes the second scrub nurse, as needed, to assist with the harvesting procedure.
      2. The instruments for the median sternotomy are moved to the center of the surgical table.
      3. The sterile back table is moved closer to the sterile field.
      4. The slush machine is moved closer to the sterile field.
   B. Equipment from the field is connected to the appropriate units/power supplies.
      1. Cell saver aspirating circuit
      2. Sternal saw
      3. Internal defibrillating paddles
      4. Two electrocautery pencils
         a. One for use during the conduit-harvesting procedure
         b. One for use during the median sternotomy procedure
      5. Extracorporeal table circuits
   C. Saphenous vein and radial artery harvesting
      1. The conduits are harvested by the assistant surgeon or PA at the same time the surgeon and the scrub nurse/tech are opening the chest in preparation for cardiopulmonary bypass or off-pump procedure.
      2. The amount and length of the conduits harvested is dependent on
         a. The number of arteries to be bypassed
         b. The specific coronary artery to be bypassed
         c. The size of the heart
         d. The diameter of the vein/arterial graft
      3. After the conduits are removed from their origin, they are flushed and distended with solution to check the diameter of the conduit and look for leaks.
      4. Handling of the vein conduits
         a. Conduits are stored in a bowl containing a saline solution pre-determined by the surgeon.
         b. Careful handling of the conduit is maintained.
            1. Prevents damage to the intimal layer
            2. Prevents the deposition of platelets and leukocytes on the intima
            3. Prevents contraction damage to the smooth muscle and disruption of the cellular matrix

5. Care of the conduit wounds
   a. Hemostasis is completed.
   b. Wounds are closed as soon as possible.
   c. Dressings are applied and the legs and arms are wrapped with Ace bandages.
6. Care of the conduit-harvesting instruments
   a. The second scrub nurse moves the conduit-harvesting instruments on the mayo stand to the periphery of the room.
   b. A sterile drape sheet is positioned over the legs and arms.
   c. The conduit-harvesting instruments remain sterile until the patient is weaned from cardiopulmonary bypass, if used, and is stable.
7. The first scrub nurse/tech moves the mayo stand with the chest instruments over the bottom of the patient's legs.

D. Internal mammary harvesting
   1. The IMA is harvested after the chest has been opened with the sternal saw.
      a. The first scrub nurse/tech assists the primary surgeon with placement of the IMA retractor and the IMA harvesting.
      b. Papaverine is available on the field for the IMA.
      c. Small ligating clips are used to occlude the branches on the IMA.
      d. After the IMA has been harvested, the IMA retractor is removed from the table.

E. CPB is instituted if not an off-pump procedure
F. Myocardial protection is accomplished according to the surgeon's request.
G. The obstructed coronary arteries are identified.
H. The distal end of the vein graft or radial artery is sewn to the coronary artery using an end-to-side anastomosis.
I. The proximal end of the vein graft is distended, measured for the appropriate length, and sewn to the aorta.
J. The heart is stimulated to beat if it does not respond on its own.
   1. The cardioplegia is turned off if CPB used.
   2. Pacing wires are used if needed.
   3. Internal defibrillation is used, as needed.
   4. The patient is normothermic.
   5. The patient's potassium is normal.
K. The patient is weaned from cardiopulmonary bypass if CPB used.
L. Hemostasis is accomplished.
M. Mediastinal drainage tubes are positioned and connected to the autotransfusion pleural drainage unit, which is connected to suction.
N. The chest is reapproximated with sternal wires.

O. Sponge, needle, and instrument counts are completed.
P. The sternal incision is closed.
Q. Dressings are applied over the sternal incision and around the mediastinal drainage tubes.
R. The instruments are moved to the periphery of the room.
  1. The instruments and back table remain sterile until the patient leaves the surgical suite.
S. Communication is accomplished with the family and the intensive care unit.
T. All required documentation is completed.
  1. Surgical record
  2. Fluid flow sheet
  3. Perfusion record
  4. Anesthesia record
  5. ICU documentation record
  6. Cardiac surgery log
U. The patient is prepared for transport to the intensive care unit
  1. The invasive lines are transferred to a transport monitor
    a. Noninvasive monitoring equipment is removed.
    b. The urine in the bladder drainage bag is drained, measured, and documented.
      1. The bladder catheter is placed on the foot of the bed.
    c. The pleural drainage unit is assessed and disconnected from the wall suction.
    d. The patient is disconnected from the anesthesia circuit and connected to an ambu bag with supplemental oxygen running.
    e. The patient is rolled slowly to the ICU bed.
    f. The ICU is notified of the transport.
    g. The anesthesiologist, circulating nurse, and hemodynamic monitoring specialist accompany the patient to the intensive care unit.

XI. Procedure Log
  A. Daily log of cases performed
    1. Type of cardiac procedure
    2. Names of surgeons
      a. Primary surgeon
      b. Assistant surgeon
      c. PA or surgeon that harvested the conduits
    3. Name of the anesthesiologist
    4. Name of the perfusionist
    5. Names of the staff members in the room and their specific roles
      a. Hemodynamic monitoring specialist

        b. Circulating nurses
        c. Scrub nurse/tech
     6. Name of the patient
     7. Date of the procedure
     8. Procedure performed
        a. Number of arteries bypassed
        b. Types of vascular conduits used
        c. Harvesting sites of vascular graft conduits
     9. Complications
     10. Any predisposing physical problems of the patient
XII. Clinical Indicators for Evaluation
   A. Patient outcomes
      1. Infection rates
         a. Chest wound
         b. Leg wounds
      2. Variances
         a. Patient
         b. System
         c. Personnel
   B. Case management
      1. Productivity
         a. Coordinated teamwork
            1. Effective communication
         b. Staff mix
         c. Team roles and responsibilities
         d. Accountability
         e. Time management
            1. Turnover times
            2. Case preparation time
         f. Safety
            1. Patient
            2. Staff
      2. Instruments and supplies
      3. Inventory
      4. Equipment
   C. Customer satisfaction
      1. Patient
      2. Family
      3. Surgeon
   D. Education
      1. Patient
      2. Staff

E. Networking
   1. Patient
   2. Family
   3. Surgeon
   4. Anesthesiologist
   5. Cath lab
   6. Emergency department
   7. Intensive care unit
   8. Cardiac step-down unit
   9. Ancillary departments

Cardiac Valve Surgery

Valve surgery becomes necessary when the patient is severely limited in activity or has symptoms such as angina or syncope that may presage sudden death.

The three most common valve procedures are those associated with the mitral valve, the aortic valve, and the tricuspid valve.

These valves can be repaired or completely replaced with a prosthesis, depending on the underlying pathology. Nonfunctioning valves cause symptoms related to their location and type of incompetence. Valves are either stenotic or incompetent.

Valves that are stenotic impede blood flowing through the heart because of the narrowed opening, usually caused by calcium deposits.

Valves that are incompetent do not completely close, causing blood to flow retrograde, inhibiting the complete emptying or filling of the heart, decreasing the available circulating blood volume.

Patients' symptoms exhibited are directly related to the valve involved and the type and degree of incompetence.

Intraoperatively, valvular surgical candidates are shaved from the neck to midthighs bilaterally. The patient is draped, leaving the chest and femoral regions exposed. The femoral arteries must be accessible should it become necessary to insert an intra-aortic balloon or due to excessive calcium use the femoral artery for cannulation for cardiopulmonary bypass.

Intraoperative transesophageal echocardiography may be used to determine whether the valve in question can be repaired or must be replaced. A probe is passed through the esophagus after the patient is asleep before cardiopulmonary bypass. This diagnostic test can indicate the flow of the venous and arterial blood, assist in the visualization of the valve, and register pressures in the different chambers of the heart.

Two types of valves are currently in use—the mechanical and biological in both the mitral and aortic positions. The type of valve used is dependent on the patient's age and underlying physical condition, and the surgeon's preference.

Mechanical valves are reserved primarily for patients 70 years old and younger. These valves appear to be more competent over a longer period of time, providing attention to the prescribed medical regime is followed. These valves require lifelong anticoagulation therapy to prevent clot formation surrounding the valve with subsequent embolization.

Biological valves, porcine valves, have a life expectancy of 7 to 10 years. These valves are reserved for those patients over 70 years old or those who are unable or unwilling to receive anticoagulation therapy. These valves are packaged sterile in a container of formalin for preservation. Before implantation, the valve is inspected for any tissue defects and put through a rinsing process. Three bowls are filled with 300 to 500 milliliters of saline. The valve is placed on a special holder and rinsed in each bowl for 2-minute intervals, totaling 6 minutes. Special handling of the valve during the rinsing process is essential so that the valve does not come into contact with the bottom or edges of the bowl. The second scrub nurse is used for this procedure while the first scrub nurse is passing the sutures needed to hold the valve in place. The valve must be kept in saline until ready to implant to prevent the tissue from drying out. Saline is squirted gently to keep the valve tissue moist while it is being sutured into place.

Valve repairs are not done as often as replacements. Repairs can be accomplished with the placement of a few sutures or a prosthetic annuloplasty ring, depending on the degree of the defect. The annuloplasty rings do not require any special handling.

Before valve replacement/repair procedures, the inventory is checked to ensure availability. Expiration dates are noted. Valves are rotated to prevent outdates.

The type and size of the valve, location of implantation, and model and serial numbers are documented on the operative record, cardiac procedure log, and appropriate valve implantation log. The type and size of the valve are placed on the patient's requisition slip for billing purposes.

Excised valves are labeled and sent to pathology. A replacement valve is ordered.

Standard of Care: Cardiac Surgery: Valve Replacement/Valve Repair Surgery

I. Indications for Valve Replacement/Repair Procedures
   A. Congenital heart disease
   B. Acquired
      1. Rheumatic disease
      2. Degenerative valvular changes
         a. Insufficient
         b. Stenosed
II. Indications of Valvular Heart Disease
   A. Symptoms exhibited are directly related to the valve involved and the type and degree of incompetence.
      1. Congestive heart failure
      2. Syncope
      3. Shortness of breath
      4. Pulmonary hypertension
      5. Myocardial hypertrophy
III. Heart Valves Affected
   A. Aortic
   B. Mitral
   C. Tricuspid
IV. Valvular Repair Versus Replacement
   A. Reconstructed, if possible
      1. Annuloplasty rings available for repair procedures
         a. Tricuspid position
         b. Mitral position
         c. A median sternotomy is performed.
         d. Cardiopulmonary bypass is required.
         e. Anticoagulation therapy is not needed.
      2. Commissurotomy
         a. Closed
            1. Left anterolateral incision
         b. Open
            1. Supine position
            2. Cardiopulmonary bypass is required.
            3. A median sternotomy is performed.
   B. Replacement
      1. Return of symptoms after reconstruction or repair

2. Replaced when a valve cannot be reconstructed
     a. Cardiopulmonary bypass is required.
     b. A median sternotomy is performed.
  C. Diagnostic procedures
     1. Cardiac catheterization
     2. Echocardiography
     3. Transesophageal echocardiography
V. Types of Valve Implants
  A. Mechanical
     1. Used on younger patient
        a. Requires lifelong anticoagulation therapy
        b. Has a shelf life of 4 years
  B. Biological
     1. Reserved for those patients over 70 years old
     2. Used on patients who are unable or will not use anticoagulation therapy
     3. Shelf life of 4 years if stored properly
        a. Must be stored at temperatures maintained between 68°F and 80°F.
     4. The valve is packaged in formalin and must be put through a rinsing process before implantation.
        a. The rinsing process is completed according to the manufacturers' guidelines.
           1. The second scrub nurse rinses the valve.
           2. The valve's integrity is checked before the rinsing process.
           3. Three bowls are filled with saline.
           4. The valve is placed on a valve holder.
           5. The valve is rinsed 2 minutes in each bowl.
              a. The valve does not scrape the bottom or the sides of the bowl.
           6. The valve is left in a clean bowl of saline until needed.
              a. The valve is moistened with saline throughout the implantation and suturing process.
VI. Preoperative Preparation of the Patient
  A. Medical and physical assessment
  B. Preoperative diagnostic testing
  C. Preoperative lab determinations
  D. Preoperative education
  E. Signed surgical consents
  F. Valve shave prep
  G. Nursing assessment
  H. Vital signs

I. NPO
VII. Preoperative Room Preparation
   A. Circulating nurse
      1. Assists the scrub nurse/tech to gather and open the appropriate supplies needed for the case
         a. Basic heart pan of instruments
         b. Valve tray
         c. Pertinent valve sizers/annuloplasty ring sizers
            1. Aortic or mitral position
            2. Mechanical or biological valve sizers
      2. All equipment needed is accounted for and functioning.
         a. Extra space is created at the head of the bed if the transesophageal echo machine is to be used.
         b. The valve/annuloplasty inventory is checked before the start of the case.
      3. Instrument, sponge, and needle counts are completed with the scrub nurse.
      4. Saline is poured into the slush machine.
      5. The scrub nurse is given heparin and any other necessary medications for use on the field.
      6. Assists the hemodynamic monitoring specialist with fluid line and cardiac supportive drug preparation
      7. Sends for the blood from the blood bank
      8. Positions the patient on the surgical table
      9. Placement of the noninvasive monitoring equipment on the patient
      10. Places chest films on the x-ray view box
   B. Scrub nurse/tech
      1. Prepares the instrumentation and sutures needed for the surgical procedure
      2. The correct valve/annuloplasty ring sizers are available.
      3. Three bowls of saline are filled if using a biological valve.
      4. The required sponge, needle, and instrument counts are completed.
   C. Hemodynamic monitoring specialist
      1. Prepares the invasive line needed by the anesthesiologist
      2. Gathers the appropriate drugs needed by the anesthesiologist for the case
      3. Assists the anesthesiologist with the invasive line placement and induction of the patient
   D. Perfusionist
      1. Prepares the heart–lung machine

2. Runs the quality assurance checks on the stat lab equipment
3. Completes the preoperative lab determinations needed before cardiopulmonary bypass
4. Calculates the required heparin dose
VIII. Valve Replacement/Repair Positioning
   A. Supine
      1. Ulnar pads are placed around both elbows and ankles.
      2. Arms are tucked at the sides after placement of invasive monitoring lines.
      3. The legs are slightly frogged to expose the femoral area.
      4. A padded roll is placed under the shoulders.
      5. A birdcage or mayo stand is placed over the patient's head.
      6. A dispersive electrode pad is positioned on an arm, flank, lower thigh, or buttock.
      7. A blanket is placed over the lower extremities, extending from the knees to the toes.
      8. A safety strap is applied just above the knees.
IX. Noninvasive and Invasive Physiologic Monitoring
   A. Noninvasive equipment
      1. BP cuff
      2. Pulse oximeter
      3. EKG electrodes
   B. Invasive equipment
      1. Arterial line
      2. Swan-Ganz line
      3. Peripheral IV
      4. Foley catheter
X. Valve Surgical Prep
   A. Requires only one person
      1. The prep starts at the chest, working down toward the extremities, prepping to the knees.
XI. Surgical Draping
   A. The anterior chest, abdomen, and thighs to the knees are exposed.
      1. The sternal incision is isolated with towels.
      2. A towel is placed over the perineum.
      3. The femoral artery region is isolated with towels.
      4. A drape sheet is placed over the knees, extending to the foot of the bed.
      5. An extra-large plastic antimicrobial-impregnated incise drape is applied over the towels, extending from the sternal notch to the femoral area.

6. A fenestrated CV drape is positioned, with the sides of the drapes run along the edges of the surgical table.
XII. Intraoperative Procedure
   A. The scrub nurse/tech moves the mayo stand over the lower extremities.
   B. The sterile back table is moved into position by the mayo stand.
   C. The slush machine/fluid warmer is moved close to the sterile back table.
   D. The equipment from the field is connected to the appropriate units/power supplies.
      1. Cell saver aspirating circuit
      2. Sternal saw
      3. Internal defibrillating paddles
      4. Electrocautery pencil
      5. Extracorporeal table circuits
   E. CPB is instituted.
   F. Myocardial protection is accomplished according to the surgeon's request.
   G. The diseased valve is excised.
   H. The valve orifice is measured with the appropriate sizer.
   I. The circulating nurse opens the valve for the scrub nurse/tech.
      1. The appropriate type of valve
      2. The correct position
      3. The correct size
      4. The valve is rinsed at this time by the second scrub nurse if it is a biological valve.
   J. The scrub nurse/tech passes the appropriate suture to the surgeon used to secure the valve into place.
   K. The diseased valve is sent to the pathology lab as a regular tissue specimen unless otherwise specified by the surgeon.
   L. The aortotomy or atriotomy is closed.
   M. The heart is stimulated to beat if it does not respond on its own.
      1. The cardioplegia is turned off.
      2. The air in the heart is vented.
      3. Pacing wires are used if needed.
      4. Internal defibrillation is used, as needed.
      5. The patient is normothermic.
      6. The patient's potassium is normal.
   N. The patient is weaned from cardiopulmonary bypass.
   O. Hemostasis is accomplished.
   P. Mediastinal drainage tubes are positioned and connected to the auto-transfusion pleural drainage unit, which is connected to suction.
   Q. The chest is reapproximated with sternal wires.

R. The sponge, needle, and instrument counts are completed.
S. The sternal incision is closed.
T. Dressings are applied over the sternal incision and around the mediastinal drainage tubes.
U. The instruments and back table are moved to the periphery of the room.
   1. The instruments and back table remain sterile until the patient leaves the surgical suite.
V. Communication is accomplished with the family and the intensive care unit.
W. All required documentation is completed.
   1. Surgical record
   2. Fluid flow sheet
   3. Perfusion record
   4. Anesthesia record
   5. Valve log book
   6. Cardiac surgery log
   7. ICU documentation record
X. The patient is prepared for transport to the intensive care unit.
   1. The invasive lines are transferred to a transport monitor
      a. Noninvasive monitoring equipment is removed.
      b. The urine in the Foley bag is drained, measured, and documented.
      c. The pleural drainage unit is assessed and disconnected from the wall suction.
      d. The patient is disconnected from the anesthesia circuit and connected to an ambu bag with supplemental oxygen running.
      e. The patient is rolled slowly to the ICU bed.
      f. The ICU is notified of the transport.
      g. The anesthesiologist, circulating nurse, and hemodynamic monitoring specialist accompany the patient to the intensive care unit.

XIII. Procedure Log
   A. Daily log of cases performed
      1. Type of cardiac procedure
      2. Names of surgeons
         a. Primary
         b. Assistant
         c. PA or NP if applicable
      3. Name of the anesthesiologist
      4. Name of the perfusionist
      5. Names of the staff members in the room and their specific roles
         a. Hemodynamic monitoring specialist

    b. Circulating nurses
    c. Scrub nurse/tech
   6. Name of the patient
   7. Date of the procedure
   8. Procedure performed
    a. Position of valve
    b. Valve repaired or replaced
    c. Type of valve implanted
    d. Size of valve implanted
    e. Model and serial number of the valve implanted.
   9. Complications
   10. Any predisposing physical problems of the patient
XIV. Special Considerations
  A. Valve Implantation Log
   1. Patient's name
   2. Date of procedure
   3. Type of valve implanted
   4. Size of valve implanted
   5. Model and serial number of the valve
  B. The manufacturers' registration card is completed.
  C. The circulating nurse ensures that the valve is charged to the patient.
  D. The valve is reordered.
  E. Annuloplasty rings are documented, charged, and reordered the same as a valve.
XV. Clinical Indicators for Evaluation
  A. Patient outcomes
  B. Infection rate
   1. Chest infections
  C. Variances
   1. Patient
   2. System
   3. Personnel
  D. Case management
   1. Productivity
    a. Coordinated teamwork
     1. Effective communication
    b. Staff mix
    c. Team roles and responsibilities
    d. Accountability
    e. Time management
     1. Turnover times

       f. Safety
          1. Patient
          2. Staff
    2. Instruments and supplies
    3. Inventory
    4. Equipment
E. Customer satisfaction
    1. Patient
    2. Family
    3. Staff
F. Education
    1. Patient
    2. Staff
G. Networking
    1. Patient
    2. Family
    3. Surgeon
    4. Anesthesiologist
    5. Cath lab
    6. Emergency department
    7. Intensive care unit
    8. Cardiac step-down unit
    9. Ancillary departments

Standard of Care: Cardiac Surgery: Cardiothoracic Procedures

I. Indications for Cardiothoracic Procedures
   A. Emergent
      1. Trauma
         a. Affecting the ascending aorta
         b. Affecting the descending aorta
   B. Scheduled
      1. Aneurysms
         a. Ascending thoracic aneurysms
         b. Descending thoracic aneurysms
   C. Medial degeneration
      1. Marfan's syndrome
II. Presenting Symptoms
   A. Symptoms indicate a compromise in circulation and/or rupture.
      1. Shock
      2. Severe pain
      3. Sudden hemorrhage
III. Special Considerations Pertaining to Ascending Thoracic Surgery
   A. Femoral bypass
      1. The enlarged and weakened aorta cannot be cannulated.
         a. Femoral artery/femoral vein
         b. Femoral artery/right atrium
            1. Femoral bypass cannot adequately drain venous return from the upper body. The right atrium is cannulated after control of the aneurysm has been accomplished.
   B. Supplies
      1. Felt sheets
      2. Aortic valve conduits
      3. Femoral perfusion cannulas
         a. Arterial
         b. Venous
      4. Extracorporeal "Y" circuit
         a. Right atrial cannula
      5. Thrombin/Gelfoam/Avitene
      6. K-thermia blanket, if requested
         a. Profound hypothermia with exsanguination may be needed.
      7. Angiograms
      8. Double-lumen endotracheal tube
   C. Instrumentation

1. Basic heart instruments
2. Valve instruments
3. Vein-harvesting/coronary artery bypass instruments
4. Femoral cannulation instruments
   D. Blood/blood products
   1. Blood
   2. Fresh frozen plasma
   3. Platelets
   E. Position
   1. Supine
   2. CABG standard of care
   F. CABG surgical prep
   1. Vein harvesting might become necessary if the dissection includes the coronary arteries
      a. Bental procedure
IV. Special Considerations Pertaining to Descending Thoracic Procedures
   A. Bypass
   1. Femoral bypass
   2. Gott shunt
   B. Supplies
   1. Femoral perfusion cannulas
      a. Arterial
      b. Venous
   2. Thrombin/Gelfoam/Avitene
   3. Angiograms
   4. Straight arterial grafts
   5. Felt sheets
   6. Double-lumen endotracheal tube
   C. Instrumentation
   1. Femoral cannulation instruments
   2. Cardiac thoracic tray
   3. An extra set of long vascular clamps
   4. Alligator clips
   5. Internal defibrillating paddles
   D. Blood/blood products
   1. These patient may exsanguinate at any moment.
      a. Blood
      b. Fresh frozen plasma
      c. Platelets
      d. Albumin, 25%
   E. Equipment
   1. Rapid volume fluid infusor/warmer and delivering unit
   2. Pressure bags

- F. Position
  1. Left posterolateral
     a. Cardiothoracic positioning standard of care
- G. Surgical prep
  1. Posterolateral chest to the knees
- H. A dispersive electrode pad is placed on the left buttock or left arm.
- I. A blanket is placed over the lower extremities, extending from the knees to the toes.
- J. A safety strap is applied across the buttock.

V. Preoperative Preparation of the Patient
   - A. Medical and physical assessment
   - B. Preoperative diagnostic testing
   - C. Preoperative lab determinations
   - D. Preoperative education
   - E. Signed surgical consents
   - F. Nursing assessment
   - G. Vital signs
   - H. NPO

VI. Preoperative Room Preparation
   - A. Circulating nurse
     1. Assists the scrub nurse/tech to gather and open the appropriate supplies needed for the case
        a. Cardiac thoracic tray
        b. Femoral cannulation tray
        c. Extra vascular clamps
     2. All equipment needed is accounted for and functioning
        a. The graft inventory is checked before the start of the case.
     3. Instrument, sponge, and needle counts are completed with the scrub nurse.
     4. Saline is poured into the slush machine and turned to the warming mode.
     5. The scrub nurse is given heparin and any other necessary medications for use on the field.
        a. Heparin is not needed if a Gott shunt is used.
     6. Assists the hemodynamic monitoring specialist with fluid line and cardiac supportive drug preparation
     7. Sends for the blood from the blood bank
     8. Positions the patient on the surgical table
     9. Placement of the noninvasive monitoring equipment on the patient
     10. Places chest films and angiograms on the x-ray view box

B. Scrub nurse/tech
   1. Prepares the instrumentation and sutures needed for the surgical procedure
   2. Long vascular clamps are readily available.
      a. The scrub nurse must be able to react quickly and efficiently in an emergency.
   3. The required sponge, needle, and instrument counts are completed.
C. Hemodynamic monitoring specialist
   1. Prepares the invasive line needed by the anesthesiologist
   2. Gathers the appropriate drugs needed by the anesthesiologist for the case
   3. Assists the anesthesiologist with the invasive line placement and induction of the patient
D. Perfusionist
   1. Prepares the heart–lung machine
   2. Runs the quality assurance checks on the stat lab equipment
   3. Completes the preoperative lab determinations needed prior to cardiopulmonary bypass
   4. Calculates the required heparin dose, if applicable

VII. Noninvasive and Invasive Physiologic Monitoring
   A. Noninvasive equipment
      1. BP cuff
      2. Pulse oximeter
      3. EKG electrodes
   B. Invasive Equipment
      1. Arterial line
      2. Swan-Ganz line
      3. Peripheral IV
      4. Foley catheter

VIII. Surgical Draping
   A. The posterolateral chest, abdomen, and thighs to the knees are exposed.
      1. The left posterolateral incision site is isolated with towels.
      2. A towel is placed over the perineum.
      3. The femoral artery region is isolated with towels.
      4. A drape sheet is placed over the knees, extending to the foot of the bed.
      5. An extra-large plastic antimicrobial-impregnated incise drape is applied over the towels, extending from the left shoulder to the femoral area.
      6. A fenestrated CV drape is positioned, with the sides of the drapes run along the edges of the surgical table.

IX. Case Progression
   A. The scrub nurse/tech moves the mayo stand over the lower extremities
      1. A second mayo stand may be needed if cannulation of the femoral artery and veins is done simultaneously with opening the chest.
   B. The sterile back table is moved into position by the mayo stand.
   C. The slush machine/fluid warmer is moved close to the sterile back table.
   D. The equipment from the field is connected to the appropriate units/power supplies.
      1. Cell saver aspirating circuit
      2. Internal defibrillating paddles
      3. Electrocautery pencil with an extension blade
      4. Extracorporeal table circuits
   E. The thoracic aorta is dissected and exposed.
   F. Femoral bypass/Gott shunt is instituted.
   G. The surgeon requests the size graft needed.
   H. The circulating nurse opens the graft for the scrub nurse/tech.
      1. The appropriate type of graft
      2. The correct size of the graft
   I. The distal and proximal ends of the thoracic aorta are clamped.
   J. The scrub nurse/tech passes the appropriate suture to the surgeon to be used to secure the graft in place.
   K. The diseased portion of the aorta is sent to the pathology lab as a regular tissue specimen unless otherwise specified by the surgeon.
   L. Alligator clips are used if needed.
   M. Internal defibrillation is used, as needed.
   N. The patient is weaned from cardiopulmonary bypass.
   O. Hemostasis is accomplished.
   P. Mediastinal drainage tubes are positioned and connected to the autotransfusion pleural drainage unit, which is connected to suction.
   Q. The chest is reapproximated with heavy suture.
   R. The sponge, needle, and instrument counts are completed.
   S. The posterolateral incision is closed.
      1. The femoral incisions are closed.
   T. Dressings are applied over the posterolateral incision and around the mediastinal drainage tubes.
   U. The instruments and back table are moved to the periphery of the room.
      1. The instruments and back table remain sterile until the patient leaves the surgical suite.
   V. Communication is accomplished with the family and the intensive care unit.

      W. All required documentation is completed.
          1. Surgical record
          2. Fluid flow sheet
          3. Perfusion record
          4. Anesthesia record
          5. Cardiac surgery log
          6. ICU documentation record
X. Transfer of the Patient
    A. The patient is prepared for transport to the intensive care unit.
        1. The invasive lines are transferred to a transport monitor.
            a. Noninvasive monitoring equipment is removed.
            b. The urine in the Foley bag is drained, measured, and documented.
            c. The pleural drainage unit is assessed and disconnected from the wall suction.
            d. The patient is disconnected from the anesthesia circuit and connected to an ambu bag with supplemental oxygen running.
            e. The patient is rolled slowly to the ICU bed.
            f. The ICU is notified of the transport.
            g. The anesthesiologist, circulating nurse, and hemodynamic monitoring specialist accompany the patient to the intensive care unit.
XI. Procedure Log
    A. Daily log of cases performed
        1. Type of cardiac procedure
        2. Names of surgeons
            a. Primary
            b. Assistant
            c. PA or NP if applicable
        3. Name of the anesthesiologist
        4. Name of the perfusionist
        5. Names of the staff members in the room and their specific roles
            a. Hemodynamic monitoring specialist
            b. Circulating nurses
            c. Scrub nurse/tech
        6. Name of the patient
        7. Date of the procedure
        8. Procedure performed
            a. Type of graft implanted
            b. Size of graft implanted
            c. Lot and serial numbers of the graft implanted

        9. Complications
      10. Any predisposing physical problems of the patient
XII. Clinical Indicators for Evaluation
    A. Patient outcomes
    B. Variances
       1. Patient
       2. System
       3. Personnel
    C. Case management
       1. Productivity
          a. Coordinated team work
             1. Effective communication
          b. Responsiveness and effectiveness in an emergency situation
          c. Team roles and responsibilities
       2. Safety
          a. Patient
          b. Staff
       3. Instruments and supplies
       4. Inventory
       5. Equipment
       6. Education
          a. Patient
          b. Staff
    D. Networking
       1. Patient
       2. Family
       3. Surgeon
       4. Anesthesiologist
       5. Cath lab
       6. Emergency department
       7. Intensive care unit
       8. Ancillary departments

Cardiac Surgery: Policy: Internal Defibrillation

Cardiac surgery's policy is the following:

1. Internal defibrillation is available for all cardiac surgical procedures.
2. Internal defibrillation paddle cords are connected to the defibrillator from the beginning of the case and for its duration. Paddles are on the field and ready for use.
3. Internal defibrillation is carried out by the physician only.
4. The staff is trained in the proper use of the defibrillator along with the corresponding power setting required for internal defibrillation.
5. External defibrillation pads with the defibrillating cable adaptors are used for repeat cardiac surgical procedures when internal defibrillation is not possible.

Cardiac Surgery: Nursing Procedure: Preparation for the Use of Internal Defibrillation

Quality Outcome: Preliminary preparation is accomplished to prepare adequately for internal defibrillation if it becomes necessary during a cardiac surgical procedure.

Performed by: Circulating nurse, scrub nurse, and surgeon

General Statement: Internal defibrillating paddles appropriate for the size of the patient are connected to the defibrillator from the beginning of the procedure until completion. The internal paddles and cords are positioned on the sterile field for quick access should it become necessary.

Equipment: Internal defibrillator cords and appropriate size for the patient and defibrillator

Steps:	Rationale:
1. Sterile paddles are opened on the sterile field	The paddle size depends on the size of the patient and the physician's preference.
2. After draping is completed, the scrub nurse hands off the end of the defibrillating cord to the circulating nurse.	The cord is connected to the defibrillator.
3. The circulating nurse turns the defibrillator to the "on" position, checking the electrical connection. The green battery-charging light is on. The button is turned "off" to the synchronizer circuit.	Ensures that the electrical connection is intact, and the defibrillator is not running off of the battery. The asynchronous circuit on the defibrillator is used for internal defibrillation.
4. If internal defibrillation becomes necessary, the scrub nurse hands the paddle handles to the surgeon. The surgeon is asked the amount of joules he or she requires.	Internal defibrillation is carried out by the physician only. Minimal current is needed when the paddles are placed directly on the heart.

Steps:	Rationale:
5. The circulating nurse sets the requested joule setting on the panel of the defibrillator when notified by the surgeon. The charge button is activated on surgeon request.	Myocardial damage resulting from defibrillatory efforts is in direct proportion to the energy used. Maximal settings, when not required, may increasingly impair an already damaged myocardium.
6. All members standing at the sterile field are notified to "clear" during defibrillation.	When using a defibrillator, neither the person holding the electrodes nor anyone else should touch the metal operating table or the patient while the current is applied to avoid self-electrocution.
7. Internal paddles are kept sterile until the patient is transferred to the intensive care unit.	Sterile supplies and instrumentation are not contaminated until the patient is safely transferred.
8. There is a sterile set of internal paddles kept in the surgical suite at times.	Emergency equipment must be available at all times.

Nursing Procedure: Preparation for the Use of Internal Defibrillation

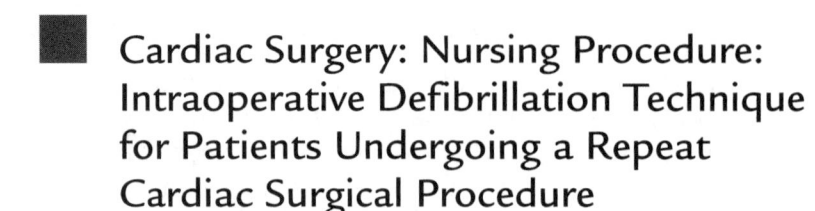

Cardiac Surgery: Nursing Procedure: Intraoperative Defibrillation Technique for Patients Undergoing a Repeat Cardiac Surgical Procedure

Quality Outcome: Defibrillation is accomplished, as needed, intraoperatively, by using externally placed defibrillating electrode pads without interruption to the integrity of the sterile field.

Performed by: Circulating nurse, anesthesiologist, and hemodynamic monitoring specialist

General Statement: Patients returning for repeat cardiac surgical procedures may have mediastinal adhesions that prevent the use of internal defibrillating paddles should defibrillation become necessary intraoperatively. Until the adhesions are dissected, these external defibrillating pads and cable adaptor provide a safe, effective method for defibrillation intraoperatively should the need arise. The defibrillator watt dial is adjusted according to physician preference and patient's response to defibrillation. The joule range using these electrode defibrillatory pads is 10 to 200 watts.

Equipment: External defibrillating electrode pads and defibrillator cable adaptor

Steps:	Rationale:
1. The circulating nurse verifies the repeat surgery status.	Adhesions surrounding the myocardium prevent the use of internal paddles for defibrillation.
2. After induction, the circulating nurse and monitoring specialist position the external defibrillating pads on the patient. The larger electrode pad is positioned behind the back, below the right scapula. The smaller electrode pad is placed laterally, below the left nipple.	This anterior–posterior position allows for more energy through the heart with optimum exposure of the surgical site.
3. The cable adaptor is connected to the electrode pads and then to the defibrillator outlet.	Proper connections are made to facilitate use without delay should it become necessary.

Steps:	Rationale:
4. The power to the defibrillator is turned on. The asynchronous circuit is selected. The defibrillator is not charged until needed.	The equipment is connected and ready for use. The asynchronous circuit is used for defibrillation. The defibrillator is not charged until needed to prevent accidental discharge and injury to staff or patient.
5. Should defibrillation become necessary intraoperatively before the release of the mediastinal from adhesions, the circulating nurse asks the physician the joules required and the defibrillator is charged. The joule range is 10 to 200 watts.	Myocardial damage resulting from defibrillatory efforts is in direct proportion to the energy used.
6. All members standing at the sterile field are notified to "clear" away from the field.	All persons must stand back from the surgical table to avoid receiving a fatal shock.
7. The circulating nurse, anesthesiologist, or hemodynamic monitoring specialist discharge the electrode pads by pushing the discharge button on the defibrillator.	The defibrillator delivers the electrical current to the patient through the electrode pads.
8. The externally placed electrode pads are removed before transfer of the patient to the intensive care unit. The sites of the electrode placement are assessed.	The skin is assessed for electrical burns.

Standard of Care: Cardiac Surgery: Defibrillation

I. Assessment of Need for Defibrillation
   A. Type of rhythm
   B. Arterial pressure
   C. Pulse
   D. Level of consciousness
   E. Predisposing factors related to ventricular irritability
II. Types of Defibrillation Techniques
   A. External
      1. Paddle handles placed over the external chest used as needed before the mediastinum is opened
      2. Externally placed electrode pads are used after the mediastinum is opened when adhesions prevent the use of internal paddles.
   B. Internal
      1. Paddle tips correspond to the size of the patient and physician's preference and are placed directly on the myocardium.
III. Safety
   A. Staff education
      1. BCLS and ACLS certified
      2. Knowledgeable of defibrillator function and care
         a. Instruction manuals available
         b. Skills checklist for every staff member
         c. Routine maintenance performed
      3. Technique for internal and external defibrillation
         a. Externally placed paddles
            1. Indications for use
            2. Appropriate position and joule range
         b. Externally placed defibrillatory electrode pads
            1. Indications for use
            2. Appropriate position and joule range
         c. Internal defibrillation
            1. Indications for use
            2. Carried out by the physician only
            3. Appropriate joule range
         d. Variables that may affect defibrillation
            1. Body weight
            2. Paddle position
            3. Electrical waveform
      4. Resistance to electrical current flow

        5. Temperature
        6. Chemical balance
           a. Electrolytes
           b. pH buffering
        7. Manipulation of the heart
        8. Hypovolemia

IV. Documentation
    A. Documentation of the type of defibrillation required
        1. Joules used to convert the cardiac dysrhythmia successfully
        2. The patient's response
    B. CPR documentation sheet completed if applicable
    C. Variance report

V. Clinical Indicators for Evaluation
    A. Staff education
        1. Time between recognition of the need for defibrillation and the response
    B. Restoration of an effective cardiac rhythm
    C. Patient safety
        1. Patient burns
    D. Staff safety
    E. Mortalities

■ Cardiac Surgery: Policy: Transfer of the Postoperative Cardiac Surgical Patient

Cardiac surgery's policy is that the following criteria be met while transporting the patient to the intensive care unit but not limited to:

1. The intensive care unit is notified when cardiopulmonary bypass has been completed with an estimated time of transfer.
2. The patient is transferred from the surgical table to the ICU bed.
3. A transport monitor is used to measure the patient's blood pressure, heart rate, rhythm, and oxygen saturation.
4. The anesthesiologist, hemodynamic monitoring specialist, and circulating nurse accompany the transfer of the patient to the intensive care unit.
5. A written and verbal report of the patient's current physical status and intraoperative events is given to the intensive care nurse.

Cardiac Surgery: Nursing Procedure: Transfer of the Postoperative Cardiac Surgical Patient

Quality Outcome: Continuity of care is provided to the cardiac surgical patient during the transition between the perioperative phase and the immediate postoperative phase.

Performed by: Cardiac anesthesiologist, hemodynamic monitoring specialist, and circulating nurse

General Statement: Written and verbal communication between cardiac surgery and the intensive care unit regarding the patient's current physical condition is accomplished to facilitate the postoperative plan of care.

Equipment: Transport monitor, EKG electrodes, transducer cable, pulse oximeter cord, ambu bag, and oxygen tank

Steps:	Rationale:
1. After cardiopulmonary bypass has been discontinued and the patient is stabilized, the circulating nurse or hemodynamic monitoring specialist telephones a verbal report of the patient's physical status and operation performed to the intensive care unit. The circulating nurse relays the approximate time of arrival to the unit.	The intraoperative course of events is communicated to the nurse recovering the cardiac patient to facilitate the postoperative plan of care. Time of arrival assists the intensive care unit with planning staffing needs to accommodate the patient.
2. The intensive care unit sends the bed to surgery prepared for transport with an oxygen tank and ambu bag attached.	The patient is placed directly on an ICU bed so that the patient is moved only once, decreasing the risk of pulling invasive lines out prematurely.

Steps:	Rationale:
3. After the sternal dressings are in place, the hemodynamic monitoring specialist and the circulating nurse transfer the EKG, pulse oximeter, and arterial line to the transport monitor to prepare the patient for transport. The transport monitor is placed at the foot of the bed.	The patient's hemodynamics are continuously monitored.
4. The hemodynamic monitoring specialist and the circulating nurse remove the noninvasive monitors.	Once the invasive lines have been transferred to the transport monitor, it is safe to disconnect the noninvasive monitoring equipment.
5. The fluid lines are transferred to the I.V. pole on the ICU bed.	All lines are transferred to the bed before moving the patient from the surgical table to prevent them from becoming dislodged.
6. The anesthesiologist disconnects the endotracheal tube from the breathing circuit on the anesthesia machine. The endotracheal tube is connected to the ambu bag with the oxygen running between 5 and 10 liters per minute.	Optimal ventilation is maintained during transport until the patient can be reconnected to a ventilator in the intensive care unit.
7. The circulating nurse assesses the amount and color of the fluid collected in the pleural drainage unit. If there are large amounts of fluid collected in the reservoir, the surgeon is notified before the patient is transferred to the intensive care bed. If there is minimal drainage, the reservoir is disconnected from suction and placed at the foot of the bed.	Large amounts of fluid collected in the reservoir could indicate postoperative hemorrhage. The pleural drainage unit is connected to suction until ready to transport to decrease the chance of fluid accumulating in the mediastinum with ensuing cardiac tamponade.

Steps:	Rationale:
8. The urine in the Foley catheter is drained, measured, and documented. The Foley catheter is positioned on the patient's leg and taped. The Foley drainage bag is hung at the foot of the bed.	Urine output is documented to be able to assess the patient's fluid needs, kidney function, and cardiac output. The Foley catheter is taped to a leg to prevent the tubing from being pulled out.
9. The circulating nurse completes the written patient transfer report and tapes it to the foot of the intensive care bed.	The documentation sheet facilitates the postoperative plan of care.
10. The patient is slowly transferred to the intensive care bed from the surgery table with a roller. The circulating nurse ensures that there are enough staff members to safely transfer the patient.	A sudden change in positioning may cause hemodynamic instability in the immediate postoperative patient. The patient is transferred slowly and with enough assistance to prevent dislodgement of the invasive lines.
11. The intensive care unit is notified of the immediate transport.	The intensive care staff is ready to receive the patient.
12. After arrival in the intensive care unit, the hemodynamic monitoring specialist assists the intensive care nurse to transfer the invasive line monitoring from the transport monitor to the unit monitor.	The patient's hemodynamics are continuously monitored. Continuity of care is provided.
13. The circulating nurse removes the pleural drainage unit from the end of the bed, places it on the floor or holder, and connects the reservoir to suction.	Suction is maintained on the pleural drainage unit to facilitate lung reexpansion and mediastinal drainage and lower the risk of pericardial tamponade.

Nursing Procedure: Transfer of the Postoperative Cardiac Surgical Patient

Steps:	Rationale:
14. The circulating nurse responds to any concerns that the intensive care nurse might have regarding the patient.	Continuity of patient care is achieved.
15. The hemodynamic monitoring specialist returns the transfer monitor to the cardiac surgery unit. The transfer monitor is plugged into an electrical source.	The transport monitor's battery is recharged so that it is functional and available at all times.

Standard of Care: Cardiac Surgery: Transfer of the Postoperative Cardiac Surgical Patient

I. Prioritizing Care
   A. Stabilization of the patient
      1. Hemostasis
      2. Physiologic stability
      3. Transfer of the patient to the intensive care bed
   B. Dressing placement
      1. Surgical incision sites
      2. Invasive line insertion sites
   C. Securing lines
   D. Transfer of monitoring equipment
      1. Continuous hemodynamic monitoring
   E. Communication
      1. Intensive care unit
      2. Family
      3. Team members
   F. Documentation
   G. Case management

II. Stabilization of the Patient
   A. Hemostasis
      1. The pleural drainage unit is connected to suction.
         a. The amount and color of the fluid in the reservoir are assessed.
            1. The surgeon is notified of excessive drainage.
            2. The incision sites are dry.
               a. Saturated dressings are redressed and brought to the attention of the surgeon.
   B. Physiologic stability
      1. Adequate cardiac output
      2. Adequate rhythm and heart rate
      3. Normothermic
         a. The patient is covered with warm blankets.
      4. Acceptable blood pressure
      5. No evidence of hemorrhage
      6. Good ventilation
         a. The endotracheal tube is secured.
         b. The patient is disconnected from the anesthesia circuit and connected to an ambu bag with supplemental oxygen.

III. Dressing Placement
    A. Surgical incision sites
        1. Sternal
        2. Leg wounds
        3. Chest tube sites
        4. Temporary pacing electrode sites
    B. Invasive line sites
        1. Arterial line
        2. Swan-Ganz line
        3. Peripheral IV line
        4. Intra-aortic balloon, if applicable

IV. Securing and Transfer of Invasive Lines
    A. Securing lines
        1. Invasive lines are secured in position with sutures or tape.
            a. Lines are positioned to permit optimal functional capacity and safety.
        2. Chest tube connections are taped.
        3. The Foley catheter is taped to the leg.
    B. Transfer of lines
        1. Invasive lines are moved to the IV pole on the intensive care bed.
        2. EKG electrodes are positioned on the patient.
            a. The EKG tracing is transferred from the surgical suite monitor to the transport monitor.
            b. The arterial transducer is recalibrated to adapt to the transport monitor.
        3. The Foley catheter drainage bag is hung at the foot of the intensive care bed.
            a. The urine is drained, measured, and documented.
        4. The pleural drainage unit is positioned at the foot of the intensive care bed.
        5. The electrocautery dispersive pad(s) is removed and the placement site(s) assessed.
        6. Temporary pacing wires
            a. If pacing, the generator is positioned on the intensive care bed to prevent tension on the temporary electrodes during the transfer.
            b. If pacing is not necessary, the temporary pacing electrodes are disconnected from the pulse generator.

V. Communication
    A. Team
        1. Individualized roles to expedite the transfer process

  2. Constant awareness of the patient's hemodynamic stability
  3. Ancillary help to assist with the transfer
 B. Intensive care unit
  1. Verbal report
   a. Procedure performed
   b. Location of invasive lines
   c. Hemodynamic stability
   d. Current cardiac-supportive drug therapy
   e. Ventilator parameters
   f. Approximate transfer time
   g. The presence of any ventricular assist devices
   h. Special considerations
  2. Written
   a. Intensive care documentation sheet
    1. Including, but not limited to
     a. Procedure performed
     b. Location of invasive lines
     c. Hemodynamic stability
     d. Current cardiac supportive drug therapy
     e. Ventilator parameters
     f. Approximate transfer time
     g. The presence of any ventricular assist devices
     h. Special considerations
 C. Family
  1. Current status of the patient
  2. The time of expected transfer to the intensive care unit
VI. Documentation
 A. Completion of the surgical report
 B. Completion of the perfusion record
 C. Completion of the anesthesia record
 D. Completion of the intensive care documentation sheet
VII. Case Management
 A. Case integrity
  1. Instrumentation remains sterile
 B. Room integrity
  1. Surgical table remains intact.
  2. Equipment remains functional.
VIII. Clinical Indicators for Evaluation
 A. Efficiency of continual monitoring
 B. Safe transfer
  1. Invasive lines remain intact.

      2. The patient remains hemodynamically stable.
- C. Availability of an intensive care unit bed
- D. Pertinent communication
  1. Continuity of care is maintained.
- E. Preparedness of room, equipment, and supplies

Special Procedures — chapter 9

Percutaneous Transluminal Coronary Angioplasty and Coronary Stenting

Percutaneous transluminal coronary angioplasty (PTCA) and coronary stenting is a nonsurgical approach to remove the obstruction in the coronary artery. This is an invasive procedure performed in the cardiac catheterization laboratory.

The basic idea of PTCA is to position a small inflatable balloon within the narrowed section of the coronary artery. Inflation of the balloon catheter causes the balloon to push outward against the narrowed wall of the artery, reducing the obstruction and increasing the blood flow to the myocardium through the coronary artery. Coronary stenting involves placement of a small stent within the lumen of the coronary artery, compressing the plaque, thereby increasing the lumen of the previously narrowed coronary artery, increasing blood flow to the myocardium. Invasive lines are placed so that the patient can be hemodynamically monitored throughout the procedure.

Both procedures may require cardiac surgical team standby support. If a "formal surgical standby" is required, scheduling this procedure is coordinated with the cardiac surgical team to ensure the availability of the cardiac surgical suite and cardiac team. The cardiac surgical team must be on-site, ready to perform emergency surgery if immediate revascularization of the myocardium becomes necessary. The patient scheduled for a PTCA or coronary stenting may sign a consent for PTCA/coronary stenting and emergency coronary artery bypass surgery.

Complications of these procedures include the following:

A. Increased chest pain and anxiety
B. Perforation of the coronary artery wall
C. Dislodgement of the coronary plaque with further obstruction or embolus

D. Arrhythmias
E. Myocardial oxygen deprivation with specific S-T segment changes leading to infarction
F. Death

Patients may reobstruct at any time after the initial dilating attempt or stenting, necessitating further evaluation with surgery or a repeat PTCA/stent procedure.

The immediate care of the patient to surgery from the cath lab is dependent on the patient's immediate hemodynamic status.

Standard of Care: Cardiac Surgery: PTCA, Coronary Stenting, and Atherectomy Surgical Support

I. Scheduling
   A. The procedure is scheduled with the surgery office and cardiac surgery manager.
      1. Date and time of surgical backup support needed
      2. Cardiologist performing the procedure
      3. Risk or rating of the procedure
      4. Coronary arteries involved
         a. Single vessel
         b. Multiple vessels
         c. Vein grafts
   B. Availability of the designated surgical suite is confirmed.
   C. The cardiac team members are notified.
      1. Date and time of procedure
      2. Any special patient considerations
         a. Dilation of vein grafts
II. Team Responsibilities During the PTCA/Coronary Stenting/Atherectomy Coverage
   A. All team members are present during the entire procedure until the clear sign is received from the cardiac catheterization lab.
   B. The cardiac surgical suite is prepared for the possibility of an emergent revascularization procedure.
      1. The supplies and instruments needed for a CABG procedure are in the cardiac surgical suite.
         a. The case supplies are not opened until the team is given notification that the patient requires emergency surgery.
         b. The supplies are organized so that they can be opened quickly.
      2. Perfusion supplies are available, but not opened.
         a. The perfusion circuit for cardiopulmonary bypass is not set up until the team is given notification that the patient requires emergency surgery.
      3. All equipment is available, inspected, and connected to power sources.
III. Patients Requiring Emergent Cardiac Surgical Revascularization
   A. Surgery notification from the catheterization lab
      1. Condition of patient
         a. Stable
         b. Unstable

2. Arrival time of the patient to surgery
3. Invasive lines present and their location
   a. Arterial line
   b. Swan-Ganz catheter
   c. Foley catheter
   d. Coronary perfusion catheter
   e. Pacing catheters
4. Cardiac supportive drug therapy instituted
   a. Type of drug
   b. Drug dose
   c. Rate of infusion
5. Mechanical assist devices present
   a. Ventilator/ambu bag
   b. Intra-aortic balloon
   c. CPR in progress
6. Special patient considerations
   a. Allergies
   b. Patient refusal of blood or blood products
   c. Fear
   d. Pain
7. Blood availability
   a. Blood typed and cross-matched

B. Facilitation of surgical intervention, intraoperative priorities
1. Quick nursing physical assessment
   a. The perioperative plan of care is reassessed as changes in the patient's hemodynamic status occur.
2. Surgical positioning of the patient
3. Noninvasive monitoring equipment applied while invasive lines are being inserted
4. Emotional support provided
5. Temperature control is supported with the use of extra blankets, as needed.
6. Pain control is provided.
7. Surgical shave prep is completed.
8. Dispersive electrode pads are positioned.
9. Surgical prep is initiated.
10. Surgeons are scrubbed.

IV. Special Considerations
A. Expedite the initiation of cardiopulmonary bypass
1. If CPR is in progress
   a. CPR is not interrupted until cardiopulmonary bypass is initiated or the patient is successfully resuscitated.

        2. Cardiopulmonary bypass may be initiated through the femoral artery and vein.
           a. The femoral cannulation tray is available.
           b. Femoral arterial and venous perfusion cannulas are available.
    B. Anticipation of additional cardiac supportive drugs (ACLS protocols)
        1. Epinephrine
        2. Levophed
        3. Lidocaine/Amiodorone
        4. Dopamine
    C. Anticipation of hemodynamic supportive devices
        1. Intra-aortic balloon pump
        2. Atrial-ventricular pacing wires and generator
        3. LVAD/RVAD
    D. Communication with the family and the intensive care unit
        1. Progress/status of the patient
        2. The estimated time of transfer to the intensive care unit
           a. Verbal and documented patient transfer report
        3. Intraoperative mortality
V. Quality Indicators for Evaluation
    A. Effective communication between the catheterization lab and cardiac surgery
    B. Team response to surgical backup notification
    C. Expedient surgical case preparation
    D. Alternative plans of care to meet the changing hemodynamic needs of the critical patient
    E. Patient outcome
        1. Safety
        2. Infection control
        3. Hemodynamic status

Cardiac Surgery: Policy: Harvesting of the Internal Mammary Artery

Cardiac surgery's policy is that the following criteria be met pertaining to the harvesting of the internal mammary artery, including but not limited to

1. IMA harvesting is at the request of the surgeon.
2. The capability to harvest an IMA is available for every CABG procedure, as needed.
3. The team members are educated in the indications, use, and special considerations associated with the harvesting of the internal mammary artery.

The Internal Mammary Artery

The left and right internal mammary arteries run along each posterior side of the sternum. The internal mammary arteries are used in conjunction with autogenous saphenous vein grafts and/or radial arteries in patients that require multiple coronary revascularizations. These arteries are felt to be the conduits of choice because of the high pressure exerted by the arterial blood flows. This high velocity helps prevent endothelial damage and thrombosis. Studies indicate that the internal mammary arteries are less susceptible to plaque formation and have the propensity to remain patent longer than saphenous veins. The adventitial pedicle is harvested along with the artery in that revascularization of the wall may occur more quickly than in the unsupported vein grafts.

Bilateral internal mammary anastomosis can be done, but the most common procedure is the use of the left internal mammary artery. This artery provides the conduit for the left anterior descending or diagonal arteries located on the anterior wall of the heart.

Consideration given to internal mammary artery harvesting is dependent on the patient's age, number and location of the obstructed coronary arteries, pulmonary function, availability and quality of the autogenous saphenous veins, and the patient's underlying physical condition.

Usually, the IMA pedicle is mobilized immediately after the sternum is divided before entering the pericardium and heparinization. A self-retaining retractor is placed in position on the left side of the table. Rakes attached to a pole(s) are placed under the sternal edge and slowly raised, lifting up on the left side of the chest for better visualization. A headlight worn by the primary surgeon and/or a special cautery pencil using a separate light source may be used to facilitate the harvesting procedure. The IMA pedicle, which consists of the IMA, the internal mammary vein, fat, muscle, and some pleura, is harvested using a diathermy cut initiated on the sternal side of the artery and vein, extending along the full length of the IMA pedicle from the sixth intercostal space to the first rib. The intercostal arteries are identified and occluded with clips on the artery side and cauterized on the chest wall side and divided. The distal end of the IMA pedicle is then divided underlying the sixth costal cartilage. After the IMA is divided, the arterial blood flow is evaluated. Papaverine is squirted on the external surface of the IMA wall and if the flow is sluggish injected into the lumen of the IMA. Papaverine helps prevent arterial spasm. The IMA is handled only as needed and with extreme care to prevent arterial spasm. The IMA is considered satisfactory if the pedicle is of good quality and the bleeding is brisk. A small bulldog is placed on the distal IMA; a moistened Ray-Tec sponge is placed over the IMA and then placed in the chest until ready for the anastomosis. If the arterial flow is not adequate, the proximal end of the IMA is divided and tied. A saphenous vein graft or radial artery is used as an alternative conduit.

After the last distal saphenous vein anastomosis is completed and an arteriotomy is made in the LAD artery, the IMA pedicle is brought into the surgical field. The anastomosis is completed with extreme care during the suturing process to prevent stenosis at the anastomosis site. The pedicle is then attached to the cardiac surface to prevent tension on the suture line. The pericardium is cut transversely on the left side to allow the pedicle to pass smoothly to the LAD artery.

Cardiac Surgery: Nursing Procedure: Harvesting of the Internal Mammary Artery

Quality Outcome: IMA harvesting is completed safely and efficiently for use as a conduit for coronary artery bypass procedures per the request of the surgeon.

Performed by: Cardiac surgeon, circulating nurses, and scrub nurses

General Statement: The primary cardiac surgeon harvests the IMA at the same time that the assistant surgeon or PA harvests the saphenous vein grafts. The left internal mammary artery is used most frequently to graft to the left anterior descending coronary artery. The right internal mammary artery can be used to graft to the right coronary artery. The mammary arteries may be used in combination with saphenous vein grafts, if multiple grafting of the coronary arteries is needed, or used by themselves if only a single vessel CABG is planned involving the RCA or the LAD artery. Bilateral mammary harvesting can also be accomplished depending upon the need of the patient and the availability of saphenous vein.

Equipment: IMA retractor, IMA table holder, papaverine, small ligating clips and appliers, electrocautery light source (optional), head light, ulnar nerve pads, and mediastinal drainage tube

Steps:	Rationale:
1. The surgeon lets the team know that an IMA is to be harvested. The surgeon specifies if it is to be a left, right, or bilateral IMA harvesting procedure.	Communication facilitates the intraoperative plan of care. The table holders for the retractor can be placed on the correct side of the table.

2. Perioperatively, the scrub nurse gathers and opens the appropriate supplies and equipment necessary for the IMA harvesting, including but not limited to
  a. IMA retractor
  b. Small ligating clips and appliers
  c. Syringe and needle
  d. Appropriate suture
  e. Electrocautery light cord, if applicable
	It is the responsibility of the scrub nurse to ensure that all the supplies needed for a cardiac case are available to prevent any unnecessary delays.

Steps:	Rationale:
3. The CABG standard of care is followed. Additional padding is placed on the patient's arm on the side of the harvesting.	Additional padding prevents the patient's arm from direct contact with the IMA bar during the harvesting procedure.
4. Before the surgical prep, the circulating nurse positions the IMA table holder on the appropriate side of the surgical table approximately at the middle of the sternum.	The IMA retractor and table holder are placed on the same side as the mammary artery to be harvested. The IMA table holder supports the IMA bar(s) used to elevate one side of the sternum.
5. The scrub nurse draws the papaverine into a syringe, with the strength and amount predetermined by the surgeon.	The papaverine is used topically on the IMA during the harvesting procedure to prevent arterial spasm.
6. After the sternum has been divided, the IMA retractor is positioned on the stabilizing bar(s). The surgeon slowly turns the crank, elevating one side of the sternum. The surgical table is raised. Good illumination is critical for the surgeon to be able to see. A head light or electrocautery pencil using a light cord may be used during the procedure.	The IMA retractor is used to raise one side of the sternum during the harvesting process. Raising the table and good illumination facilitate visualization during the harvesting.
7. The surgeon dissects out the IMA using the electrocautery. The scrub nurse has small ligating clips ready for the surgeon.	During the harvesting, the surgeon places small ligating clips on the artery side of the collateral branches.
8. After the IMA has been freed from the chest wall, sternal notch to the xiphoid, the scrub nurse gives the papaverine to the surgeon to squirt on the IMA pedicle. A mediastinal drainage tube is inserted into the affected pleura space.	The papaverine prevents arterial spasm. The pleura is opened on the side of the harvesting, and a mediastinal tube is positioned to facilitate drainage.

Steps:	Rationale:
9. After the harvesting is completed, the scrub nurse removes the IMA retractor, and the circulating nurse removes the IMA table holder and lowers the surgical table. If bilateral IMA harvesting is to be done, the stabilizing bar and the table holder are moved to the other side.	The IMA retractor is not needed again unless the surgeon is doing another IMA harvesting on the opposite side.
10. The surgeon prepares the patient for cardiopulmonary bypass or off-pump procedure.	CPB may be necessary for the revascularization process. All attempts may be made toward an off-pump procedure.
11. After implementation of cardiopulmonary bypass, the surgeon prepares the IMA by dividing the artery and tying the distal end of the vessel. The arterial flow of the vessel is checked to ensure that it is good. A small slit is made in the beveled artery. The surgeon and scrub nurse handle the pedicle only, not the artery itself.	The IMA is very susceptible to spasm and damage with improper handling. If the artery is in spasm, the arterial blood flow will be poor. The flow must be good or a vein graft will be used as a substitute.
12. A coronary arteriotomy is made and the surgeon performs a typical anastomosis. The scrub nurse has an air blower or syringe full of saline to squirt on the artery for visualization during the anastomosis. After the anastomosis, the pedicle is tacked to the epicardium.	Only the distal end of the IMA is anastomosed. The proximal end is not divided from its origin. The pedicle is tacked to the epicardium to prevent strain and subsequent tenting of the distal anastomosis. It also prevents the pedicle from adhering to the chest wall.
13. If saphenous vein grafts/radial artery grafts are also used, the IMA anastomosis is completed last.	The IMA will be stressed with the manipulation of the heart.

Steps:	Rationale:
14. Before weaning the patient from cardiopulmonary bypass, the surgeon feels the pulse in the IMA. The EKG is observed for signs of ischemia. The mean arterial blood pressure is kept around 90 mm Hg.	A mean pressure of 90 mm Hg is needed to perfuse the IMA. If the blood flow through the IMA is not sufficient, the EKG will show signs of ischemia.
15. Before placement of the sternal wires, the surgeon will position two more mediastinal drainage tubes. All three tubes are connected to the pleural drainage unit and connected to suction.	The mediastinal tubes facilitate postoperative chest drainage and re-expansion of the lungs.

Standard of Care: Cardiac Surgery: Harvesting of the Internal Mammary Artery

I. Utilization of the IMA
   A. CABG procedures
      1. Conduits used in conjunction with the saphenous vein grafts
         a. LAD artery
         b. RCA artery
      2. Conduits used instead of saphenous vein grafts
         a. LAD artery
         b. RCA artery
         c. Left and right radial arteries
II. Location of the Internal Mammary Arteries
   A. Inferior chest wall
      1. Left inferior chest wall
      2. Right inferior chest wall
III. Benefits of an IMA Versus a Saphenous Vein
   A. The long-term patency rate is increased approximately 90%.
   B. The long-term survival is improved.
   C. The incidence of myocardial infarction, hospitalization, and/or reoperation because of cardiac causes is decreased.
   D. The IMA is immune to atherosclerosis.
   E. If done as a single bypass, the absence of leg wounds greatly reduces the potential postoperative complications and eliminates postoperative leg pain.
IV. Contraindications to IMA Grafting
   A. Lack of blood supply to the mediastinum
   B. Large coronary arteries in conjunction with a hypertrophied left ventricle
   C. Extensive brachiocephalic atherosclerosis
   D. Poor flow through the IMA
V. Equipment Required for IMA Harvesting
   A. IMA retractor
      1. The IMA retractors are dependent upon surgeon preference and provide the ability to raise one side of the sternum to facilitate visualization of the IMA. Some retractors require a bar stabilization on the surgery table and applied by the circulating nurse while others are placed in position by the surgeon on the field without the need of a stabilization bar.
   B. Cautery pencil with a light source attachment (optional)

    1. Small ligating clips and appliers
    2. A syringe of papaverine
    3. An additional mediastinal chest drainage tube
VI. Intraoperative Preparation for IMA Harvesting
 A. CABG standard of care
 B. IMA table holder is positioned on the appropriate side of the table.
  1. The holder goes on the same side as the artery to be harvested.
 C. The IMA retractor is opened on the sterile field.
 D. The papaverine is drawn up in a syringe by the scrub nurse.
 E. Additional padding is necessary to protect the patient's arms from contact with the retractor stabilizing bar.
 F. The retractor is positioned on the supporting bar/bars as soon as the sternum has been divided with the sternal saw about midsternal level.
 G. The table is raised to the highest position for optimal visualization for the surgeon.
  1. The surgeon may request a stool to sit on.
 H. The surgeon dissects the IMA distally.
  1. Small ligating clips are placed on the artery side of the collateral branches.
 I. After harvesting, the IMA retractor and table holders are removed.
 J. If a bilateral IMA dissection is being done, the identical positioning and procedure are repeated on the opposite side.
 K. After institution of cardiopulmonary bypass, the surgeon prepares the IMA for the anastomosis.
  1. The IMA is divided distally.
  2. The distal IMA is tied.
  3. The surgeon prepares the end of the artery to be anastomosed.
   1. Care is taken not to manipulate the artery itself.
    a. The adventitia is grasped gently.
  4. If used in conjunction with saphenous vein grafting, the IMA anastomosis is completed last.
  5. The surgeon performs a typical coronary anastomosis with the suture of his choice.
  6. When the anastomosis is complete, the IMA pedicle is tacked to the epicardium.
  7. There is no proximal end to an IMA that needs to be anastomosed because the proximal end of the IMA is left connected to its origin.
  8. A mediastinal drainage tube is inserted into the pleura on the same side as the harvesting.
VII. Clinical Indicators for Evaluation
 A. Availability of instrumentation needed for IMA harvesting
 B. Staff education

C. Postoperative complications
   1. Infection rate
   2. IMA patency rate
   3. Postoperative pain
   4. Pulmonary complications

Cardiac Surgery: Policy: Special Procedures: Slush Machine

Cardiac surgery's policy is that a slush machine with the capability to heat or cool saline be available for all cardiac surgical procedures. Normothermia or hypothermia may be used during cardiopulmonary bypass to prolong safe operating time by minimizing ischemic damage to the heart. The decision for hypothermia or normothermia used during the cardiac procedure will come from the physician.

Cardiac Surgery: Nursing Procedure: Slush Machine

Quality Outcome: Hypothermia or normothermia techniques may be used for myocardial protection during a cardiac procedure to prolong safe operating time by minimizing ischemic damage to the heart.

Performed by: Circulating nurse and scrub nurse

General Statement: The cardiac nursing staff will have the ability to operate the slush machine in the cooling or heating mode, according to physician preference, to meet the needs of the individual patient.

Equipment: A slush machine that has the ability to heat or cool saline, a slush machine drape, normal saline (3 to 4 liters), dependent on need

Steps:	Rationale:
1. The circulating nurse confers with the surgeon on the type of myocardial protection used for the procedure.	Heating or cooling is used to facilitate myocardial protection.
2. The slush machine is available and connected to the power source.	Standard cardiac equipment is left in the cardiac surgical suite at all times.
3. The scrub nurse drapes the slush machine during preparation of the sterile field.	The drape provides a sterile barrier between the machine and the saline.
4. The circulating nurse pours 3 liters of saline into the basin of the slush machine and turns the machine on to the appropriate mode, heating or cooling.	The process to achieve the appropriate saline temperature is initiated.

Steps:	Rationale:
5. If cooling, the saline must be stirred intermittently to create slush. When the slush has reached its desired consistency, the machine is turned off. When in the warming mode, a thermometer is used to prevent the saline from reaching a higher temperature than 39° Centigrade. The machine can be turned off or cool saline can be added if the saline gets too warm.	Hard ice will form along the sides of the basin if not stirred. A temperature check using a thermometer is necessary to prevent the possibility of burns caused from saline that is too warm.
6. The circulating nurse documents the amount and type of solution utilized, along with the temperature mode.	All solutions added to the sterile field are documented. All perioperative care is documented.
7. At the end of the procedure, the scrub nurse disposes of the remaining saline and the slush drape. The machine is turned off and unplugged from its power source. The machine is wiped down with an approved disinfectant.	All equipment used during the surgical procedure is considered contaminated and should be cleaned with a hospital-grade disinfectant. The machine is disconnected from its power source to prevent inadvertent activation during the housekeeping procedures.

Cardiac Surgery: Policy: Intraoperative Preparation of the Autotransfusion Pleural Drainage Unit

Cardiac surgery's policy is that the following criteria be met when using the autotransfusion pleural drainage unit, including but not limited to

1. The manufacturer's guidelines for the preparation and use of the autotransfusion drainage system are followed.
2. The system is ordered and supervised by the attending physician.
3. Staff members are educated in the preparation and use of the autotransfusion pleural drainage unit.
4. Aseptic technique is used during all stages of the preparation and use of the system.

Cardiac Surgery: Nursing Procedure: Preparation of the Autotransfusion Pleural Drainage Unit

Quality Outcome: An autotransfusion pleural drainage unit is prepared intraoperatively to enable the collection of shed mediastinal blood, filter it, and return it to the patient safely.

Performed by: Hemodynamic monitoring specialist, circulating nurse, and scrub nurse

General Statement: The cell saver reservoir used intraoperatively for the collection of shed mediastinal blood at the surgical site can be converted to a postoperative pleural drainage unit capable of autotransfusion. The manufacturer's guidelines are followed for the preparation and use of the system. Chest drainage systems with built-in autotransfusion capabilities may also be used dependent upon physician preference.

Equipment: Collection reservoir with a water seal and manometer chamber, autotransfusion conversion kit, transport reservoir stand, and suction

Steps:	Rationale:
1. During the initial case preparation, the circulating nurse removes the collection reservoir from the packaging box and inspects the sterile bag for damage.	The sterility of the reservoir may be compromised if the package is damaged.
2. The collection reservoir is positioned on the cell saver unit for the surgical procedure. A separate autotransfusion pleural drainage unit may be used as well.	The collection reservoir is used for the collection of lost blood intraoperatively in conjunction with the cell saver unit.
3. After cessation of cardiopulmonary bypass and the patient is stabilized, the circulating nurse opens the conversion kit, removes the mediastinal drainage package, and opens it on the sterile field for the scrub nurse.	The mediastinal drainage package contains latex tubing and connectors needed to connect the mediastinal tubes to the pleural drainage unit. The patient is stabilized before the nurse opens any patient-chargeable item that may not be needed if the patient is unable to be weaned from cardiopulmonary bypass.

Steps:	Rationale:
4. When the intraoperative blood losses are at a minimum and blood in the reservoir has been spun down by the cell saver, the collection reservoir is disconnected from the cell saver.	The reservoir is converted to a pleural drainage unit.
5. The circulating nurse converts the collection reservoir to a pleural drainage unit following the manufacturer's guidelines. Strict aseptic technique is used.	Strict aseptic technique is followed for preparation and use of the entire system to prevent the chance of systemic infection spread through the blood. The drainage system prevents outside air from being drawn into the pleural space during expiration. Saline is used to fill the pleural drainage unit's water seal and manometer chambers. Fluid in the collection unit seals off outside air to maintain negative pressure within the pleural cavity.

    a. The filter bypass shunt line is positioned on the vent/vacuum port and quick prime port.
    b. Nonvented caps are placed over the four aspirating circuits.
    c. The chest drainage line port is connected to the inlet adaptor at the top of the reservoir.
    d. The micro air filter is attached to the low negative pressure relief valve.
    e. The cap lock quick-release connector is clamped shut and positioned at the bottom of the reservoir.
    f. The scrub nurse fills a 60-ml syringe full of saline and gives it to the circulating nurse.
    g. The circulating nurse fills the manometer chamber to the desired level of suction through the manometer vent, approximately 18 ml of fluid. The water seal chamber is filled to the 2-ml line.
    h. The reservoir water seal communication line is attached to the water seal chamber luer connector.
    i. All connections at the top of the reservoir are tightened. — Ensures an airtight seal.

Nursing Procedure: Preparation of the Autotransfusion Pleural Drainage Unit

Steps:	Rationale:
6. The converted reservoir is positioned at the foot of the surgical table in the transport reservoir's stand. The reservoir is kept at subthoracic levels and out of the path of traffic.	The location of the stand is positioned in close proximity to the mediastinal drainage tubing for easy connection to the reservoir and in a place where the reservoir will not inadvertently be knocked over. The collection reservoir is kept below the level of the chest to facilitate gravity drainage and prevent retrograde flow of the drainage.

7. The scrub nurse assembles the drainage line with the addition of the appropriate connectors to adapt to the chest tubes.
   a. The proximal end of the latex tubing is connected to the chest tubes.
   b. The distal end of the latex tubing is handed to the circulating nurse, who connects it to the collection reservoir. The scrub nurse ensures that the ends of the tubing being passed off are not contaminated.
	The ends of the drainage tubing remain sterile throughout the preparation process to decrease the chance of infection. Assembly of the pleural drainage system is complete.

8. The circulating nurse attaches the vacuum line to the wall suction, which is set between 30 cm and 200 cm of H_2O. The circulating nurse rotates the adjustable flow regulator until bubbling is observed in the water manometer chamber. The circulating nurse checks the suction level.	The water level in the manometer regulates the amount of vacuum delivered. The circulating nurse ensures that the level of suction is consistent with the surgeon's request and is activated as appropriate for the system being used. If the chamber is not bubbling, it might indicate a clogged or kinked mediastinal tube, not enough suction coming from the wall suction apparatus, or loose connections on the pleural drainage unit.

Steps:	Rationale:
9. The autotransfusion extension line is connected to the reservoir outlet.	This line facilitates the delivery of the filtered shed mediastinal blood back to the patient.
10. Should autotransfusion become necessary in the surgical suite, the extension outlet tubing is connected to an I.V. line; the rate and amount infused are monitored by an infusion pump according to the specific instructions of the surgeon.	Autotransfusion is ordered and supervised by the attending surgeon.
11. The scrub nurse places slit sponges around the mediastinal tubes.	Drain sites are dressed separately from the incision site to prevent contamination of the surgical wound from secretions around the drains.
12. Upon preparation for transport, the circulating nurse assesses the pleural drainage unit for the amount and color of mediastinal drainage collected. The circulating nurse ensures that there is no tension or kinks on the mediastinal drainage line during the transfer of the patient from the surgical table to the intensive care unit bed.	Excessive drainage that is bright red in color may be indicative of life-threatening hemorrhage. Tension placed on the mediastinal drainage tubing may cause the dislodgement of the mediastinal tubes or the inadvertent disconnection of the pleural drainage unit.
13. The circulating nurse positions the pleural drainage unit at the foot of the intensive care unit bed. The suction regulator is turned off, and the vacuum line is disconnected from the wall suction apparatus. Suction of the pleural drainage unit is the last item to be disconnected before transport and one of the first items to be reconnected once in the intensive care unit.	Suction on the pleural drainage unit is maintained to prevent the accumulation of mediastinal fluids within the chest with resultant cardiac tamponade.

Nursing Procedure: Preparation of the Autotransfusion Pleural Drainage Unit

Steps:	Rationale:
14. After arriving in the intensive care unit, the circulating nurse removes the pleural drainage unit from the transport holder and places it on a "C" clamp positioned on an I.V. pole at the foot of the bed.	The "C" clamp is positioned at subthoracic levels and secures the reservoir to the I.V. pole, preventing the reservoir from being knocked over.
15. The circulating nurse assists the intensive care nurse with re-establishing suction to the pleural drainage unit to facilitate the evacuation of air and fluid.	Continual suction ensures the evacuation of air and fluid from the pleural cavity.

Standard of Care: Cardiac Surgery: Intraoperative Preparation of the Autotransfusion Pleural Drainage Unit

I. Indications for Use
   A. Ordered and supervised by the attending surgeon
      1. The surgeon determines the time, rate, and volume to be transfused.
   B. Intraoperative
      1. Used on all cardiac surgical procedures
      2. Used on cardiothoracic surgical procedures where there is an increased risk of hemorrhage
   C. Postoperative
      1. Intensive care unit
         a. Pleural drainage unit
         b. Autotransfusion system

II. Benefits of the Mediastinal Autotransfusion System
   A. The system's reservoir is used intraoperatively before heparinization and after reversal of heparin to collect shed blood at the surgical site.
   B. The reservoir system is converted to a postoperative pleural drainage unit.
   C. The system collects, filters, and autotransfuses the patient's shed postoperative mediastinal blood.
   D. This decreases the need for homologous blood transfusion.
   E. This may be an acceptable form of transfusion for those patients refusing homologous blood because of religious beliefs.

III. Components of the Mediastinal Drainage System
   A. Collection reservoir
   B. Conversion kit
   C. Transport reservoir stand
   D. Suction

IV. Collection Reservoir
   A. Reservoir characteristics
      1. Integral water seal and water manometer chambers
         a. The negative pressure within the pleural cavity is re-established.
      2. Micron filter
         a. Defoams and filters shed blood and particulate matter.
      3. Volume capacity
         a. Holds 3500 ml of fluid

V. Conversion Pack Components if Converting an Autotransfusion Device

       A. Cardiotomy conversion pack
          1. Nonvented nozzle covers
          2. Micro air filter
          3. Filter bypass shunt
          4. Inlet adaptor
          5. Infusion line adaptor
          6. Vacuum line with an adjustable flow control
          7. Extension line
          8. Detachable spike adaptor
       B. Mediastinal drainage table pack
          1. Latex drainage line
          2. Straight connectors
          3. One 3/8" × 3/8" × 3/8" connector
       C. Surgeon may choose to use a single, disposable collecting chamber with built-in manometer and water seal along with an autotransfusion device

VI. Contraindications for the Use of the Autotransfusion System
       A. The presence of pulmonary, pericardial, mediastinal, or systemic infection
       B. The existence of gross contamination, malignancy, perforated intestine, or lymphatic failure
       C. The existence of gross perforations of the chest wall
       D. After the patient is returned to surgery for any reason
       E. When the mediastinum is opened and vacuum is applied

VII. Special Considerations
       A. The manufacturer's guidelines are followed for the preparation and use of the system.
       B. Aseptic technique is used during all stages of preparation and use of the system.
       C. All connections are airtight.
       D. The integrity of the collection reservoir is inspected before use.
       E. Blood collected in the reservoir must be returned to the patient within 4 hours of the collection time.
       F. Continual bubbling occurs in the manometer chamber.

VIII. Intraoperative Preparation
       A. The collection reservoir may be used as the cell saver reservoir until the sternal wires are in place and any significant bleeding is controlled. If a cell saver is not used, the surgeon may use a dual-chamber collection device with built-in manometer with autotransfusion capabilities.
       B. The reservoir is disconnected from the cell saver and placed in the transport stand.

C. The conversion pack is opened.
   1. The mediastinal drainage package is opened on the sterile field for the scrub nurse.
   2. The collection reservoir is converted to a pleural drainage system.
D. The water seal chamber is filled to the 2-ml mark.
E. The manometer is filled to the desired level of suction, approximately 18 ml.
F. The scrub nurse/tech assembles the drainage line with placement of the appropriate connectors to adapt to the chest tubes.
   1. The proximal end of the latex tubing is connected to the chest tubes.
   2. The distal end of the latex tubing is handed to the circulating nurse, who connects it to the collection reservoir.
G. The autotransfusion system line is attached to the port on the bottom of the collection reservoir.
H. Suction is applied to the vacuum port on the collection reservoir.
I. Suction is adjusted in the vacuum line until bubbling is observed in the manometer chamber.

IX. Preparation for Transport with the Autotransfusion System
   A. Assessment of the autotransfusion system
      1. All connections are checked to ensure they are secure and airtight.
      2. Continual bubbling is maintained in the manometer chamber.
         a. Bubbling in the water seal chamber indicates an air leak with the patient or in the system.
      3. The amount and color of fluid collected in the reservoir are assessed.
         a. The surgeon is notified of excessive mediastinal drainage.
      4. The mediastinal drainage tubing is checked to ensure that no unnecessary tension is placed on the line during the transfer of the patient from the surgical table to the intensive care unit bed.
   B. Positioning of the pleural drainage unit during transport
      1. The pleural drainage unit is hung at the foot of the intensive care unit bed.
      2. After the patient has been moved to the intensive care unit bed, the suction is turned off at the suction regulator valve on the suction line, and the line is then disconnected from the wall suction.

X. Preparation of the Autotransfusion System in the Intensive Care Unit
   A. The circulating nurse assists the intensive care unit nurse with the initial preparation of the autotransfusion system.
      1. The pleural drainage unit is removed from the transport stand and placed on a "C" clamp that is connected to an I.V. pole or placed on the floor.
      2. The "C" clamp is positioned on the I.V. pole at subthoracic levels.

3. The "C" clamp is attached securely to the I.V. pole.
4. The reservoir and blood collection circuits are assessed to ensure that they are positioned at subthoracic levels.
5. Suction is reapplied to the pleural drainage unit and regulated by the suction valve regulator on the aspiration line.
6. The circulating nurse ensures that there is continual bubbling in the manometer chamber.

XI. Clinical Indicators for Evaluation
   A. Efficacy of utilization
   B. Trend in bank blood utilization
   C. Complications related to the pleural autotransfusion system
   D. Staff education
      1. Initial preparation
      2. Instituting the system
      3. Postoperative autotransfusion

Cardiac Surgery: Policy: Repeat Cardiac Surgical Procedures

Cardiac surgery's policy is that the following criteria be met when preparing for a repeat cardiac surgical procedure, including but not limited to

1. The re-op procedure is indicated on the surgery schedule as a "re-operation."
2. The history of the previous cardiac surgical procedure is communicated to the cardiac team.
3. Special equipment is available for intraoperative use.
   a. External defibrillating electrode pads
   b. Oscillating saw
   c. Child chest retractor
   d. Femoral cannulation tray
   e. Femoral perfusion cannulas, arterial and venous
   f. Anterior/posterior and lateral chest films
   g. Alligator clips and pulse generator
   h. Hemostasis supplies
4. The cardiac team has an alternate plan of care devised if precipitating events warrant a change in standard operating procedure.

Preoperative communication and organization of special supplies and equipment facilitate a safe intraoperative plan of care for the patient undergoing a repeat cardiac surgical procedure. Emergency equipment is available if a change in events of patient's condition warrants advanced cardiac life support.

Cardiac Surgery: Nursing Procedure: Repeat Cardiac Surgical Procedures

Quality Outcome: An intraoperative plan of care is devised to meet the current or changing needs of the patient safely undergoing a repeat cardiac surgical procedure.

Performed by: Cardiac anesthesiologist, cardiac surgeon, perfusionist, hemodynamic monitoring specialist, circulating nurse, and scrub nurse

General Statement: Preoperative communication and organization of special supplies and equipment facilitate a safe intraoperative plan of care for the patient undergoing a repeat cardiac surgical procedure.

Equipment: External defibrillating electrode pads; oscillating saw; child chest retractor; femoral cannulation tray; femoral perfusion catheters, arterial and venous; alligator clips and pulse generator; hemostasis supplies; and chest x-rays, anterior/posterior and lateral

Steps:	Rationale:
1. The cardiac manager relays the pertinent scheduling information to the cardiac team.	The communication of the patient's previous surgery facilitates the intraoperative plan of care by the cardiac team for the patient.
2. The circulating nurse and the scrub nurse gather the necessary equipment.	The equipment is available before the excision of myocardial adhesions.
3. The team is trained to revise the intraoperative plan of care at any given moment to meet the imminent needs of the patient.	Actions are prioritized to meet the needs of the patient and surgeon.

Steps:

4. The standard of care for the specific cardiac procedure is followed with the addition of the following:
   a. After induction, the circulating nurse and the hemodynamic monitoring specialist position the external defibrillating pads on the patient.
   b. The chest films are displayed on the view box or computer screen.
   c. The scrub nurse has the femoral cannulation tray and femoral perfusion catheters available if the need arises.
   d. The scrub nurse prepares some additional pledgeted suture. Felt strips are available.
   e. Topical hemostatic agents are available if requested by the surgeon.
   f. The supply and demand of blood products are met.
   g. Communication with the intensive care unit and family is accomplished.
   h. Alligator clips and a pulse generator are available if pacing is required to facilitate safe surgical intervention.

Rationale:

The standards provide guidelines of care. The defibrillating pads provide a safe, effective method for defibrillation if needed intraoperatively, when adhesions prevent the use of internal paddles for defibrillation.

The x-rays help to visualize the space between the myocardium and the sternum, indicating the degree of sternal adhesions. Adhesion formation surrounding the myocardium may prevent cardiopulmonary bypass through the standard route. If excessive bleeding occurs before the release of the adhesions, femoral artery/vein bypass may be instituted.

Tearing of the myocardium and tissues surrounding the myocardium may occur, causing hemorrhage at the surgical site.

Re-operations require a longer surgical operating time due to adhesion formation.

Keeping the family informed reduces anxiety.

Alligator clips provide a quick method for temporary pacing in the presence of myocardial adhesions.

Cardiac Surgery: Standard of Care: Repeat Cardiac Surgical Procedures

I. Preliminary Case Preparation
   A. Scheduling
      1. Indicated on the surgery schedule as "re-operation."
      2. The cardiac manager relates case information to the cardiac team.
      3. A history of previous cardiac surgery is acquired.
         a. If previous CABG
            1. The location of any patent grafts
            2. Harvesting sites available for coronary graft conduits
         a. If previous valve repair/replacement
            1. Previous incision site
               a. Lateral chest
               b. Median sternotomy
            2. Valve/annuloplasty position
               a. Aortic
               b. Mitral
               c. Tricuspid

II. Special Equipment Needs
   A. External defibrillating electrode pads
      1. These electrode pads are applied to the back, behind the right scapula, and then laterally, below the left nipple.
   B. Oscillating saw
   C. Child chest retractor
   D. Femoral cannulation tray available
   E. Femoral perfusion cannulas
      1. Arterial
      2. Venous
   F. Anterior/posterior and lateral chest films
   G. Alligator clips and pulse generator

III. Hemostasis Considerations
   A. Pledgeted sutures available
   B. Felt sheets available
   C. Fresh frozen plasma and platelets are available on physician request after cessation of cardiopulmonary bypass.
   D. Topical hemostatic agents are available.

IV. Team Education
   A. Advanced cardiac life support
   B. Prioritizing actions of care delivered dependent upon the current status of the patient

       C. Alternate routes of cardiopulmonary bypass
V. Quality Indicators for Evaluation
    A. Number of repeat cardiac surgical procedures
    B. Pertinent scheduling information
    C. Availability of special instruments and supplies
    D. Patient outcome
       1. Safety
       2. Hemodynamic status
       3. Infection rate
       4. Intraoperative mortality rate
    E. Blood/blood product utilization
    F. Team response to emergency situations

Cardiac Surgery: Policy: Femoral Artery Cannulation

Cardiac surgery's policy is that supplies, equipment, and instrumentation be available at all times for femoral cannulation if the need arises to institute femoral cannulation for cardiopulmonary bypass or insertion of an intra-aortic balloon in response to a change in the patient's physiologic condition.

Cardiac Surgery: Nursing Procedure: Femoral Artery Cannulation

Quality Outcome: Femoral cannulation is accomplished efficiently and effectively as an alternate approach for institution of cardiopulmonary bypass when warranted by the patient's physiologic condition.

Performed by: Cardiac surgeon, perfusionist, circulating nurse, and scrub nurse

General Statement: The femoral artery and vein are used for cannulation sites for cardiopulmonary bypass if the conventional method of cannulating the aorta and right atrium is inaccessible or if warranted by the patient's condition. Dependent on the physiologic status of the patient, a second team may prepare the femoral cannulation site. If CPR is in progress during the transport of the patient to the surgical suite, priorities are aimed at facilitating cardiopulmonary bypass without interruption of CPR.

Equipment: Femoral arterial and venous perfusion cannulas, extracorporeal table circuit, and femoral cannulation tray

Steps:	Rationale:
1. The surgeon communicates the need for femoral cannulation preoperatively.	Pertinent communication enables the team to plan the intraoperative care of the patient.
2. The scrub nurse gathers and organizes the femoral cannulation supplies. If a separate team is isolating the femoral artery/vein while the surgeon is opening the mediastinum, the scrub nurse prepares a second mayo stand with the pertinent femoral equipment.	The scrub nurse is responsible for organizing and ensuring that the appropriate equipment is available before the start of the procedure. If femoral cannulation is not done on an emergent basis, a separate tray of instruments is organized to prevent cross-contamination of the surgical incision sites.
3. The circulating nurse preps the patient from the umbilicus to the knees.	The femoral region of the patient is prepped for all cardiac surgical procedures because femoral cannulation may become necessary at any time intraoperatively.

Steps:	Rationale:
4. The first scrub nurse prepares the extracorporeal table circuits for cardiopulmonary bypass. The procedure for cardiopulmonary bypass is followed.	The table circuits are ready to connect to the perfusion cannulas after they have been inserted into the femoral artery and vein to prevent unnecessary blood loss and facilitate cardiopulmonary bypass.
5. The second scrub nurse assists the surgeon in exposing and isolating the femoral artery and vein. The second scrub nurse has vascular clamps and the perfusion cannulas clamped and ready. When the perfusion catheters are inserted, the second scrub nurse hands the surgeon the appropriate extracorporeal circuit to connect to the cannula.	Umbilical tapes are placed around the artery, and vein and vascular clamps are used to maintain control of the vessel during the cannulation process. The femoral perfusion catheters do not have an occlusive cap over the distal end. A line clamp is positioned to prevent unnecessary blood loss during cannulation.
6. The second scrub nurse assists the surgeon with securing the extracorporeal circuit.	The perfusion cannulas are sewn down to prevent their accidental dislodgement during the procedure.
7. Extra suture is organized to close the femoral cannulation sites.	After cessation of cardiopulmonary bypass and the patient is stabilized, the cannulas are removed, and the femoral incisions are closed.

Standard of Care: Cardiac Surgery: Femoral Cannulation for Cardiopulmonary Bypass

I. Types of Femoral Cannulation for Cardiopulmonary Bypass
   A. Femoral artery/femoral vein cannulation
   B. Femoral artery/right atrium cannulation
   C. Femoral artery/femoral vein to right atrium cannulation
II. Indications for Femoral Artery/Femoral Vein Cannulation
   A. Ascending aortic aneurysms
   B. Cardiac surgery reoperations with sternal adhesions
   C. Transfer of the unstable cardiac surgical patient to the surgical suite, CPR in progress
   D. Thoracic aneurysms
III. Indications for Femoral Artery Cannulation
   A. Partial bypass
   B. Placement of an intra-aortic balloon when it cannot be passed percutaneously
IV. Supplies Needed for Femoral Cannulation
   A. Perfusion supplies
      1. Femoral arterial cannulas
         a. Percutaneous insertion
         b. Cutdown insertion
      2. Femoral venous cannulas
         a. Percutaneous insertion
         b. Cutdown insertion
   B. Instrumentation
      1. Femoral cannulation instruments
      2. Umbilical tapes/vessel loops
      3. Tourniquets
V. Intraoperative Procedure Considerations
   A. Emergent procedure
      1. The patient's groin is quickly prepped.
      2. Unless the case has been previously prepared, the femoral cannulation instruments are used to get on bypass.
      3. CPR is continued while the team is isolating the femoral artery and vein and preparing for cardiopulmonary bypass.
      4. After cardiopulmonary bypass is established, CPR is discontinued, the patient's chest is prepped, and the mediastinum is opened in the usual fashion.

5. Supplies and cannulation sutures are available if the need arises to change the cannulation sites from the femoral arterial/vein to the aorta or right atrium because of poor arterial flow or venous return.
  B. Scheduled femoral cannulation
    1. The femoral artery/vein is exposed at the same time the mediastinum is opened.
      a. A separate mayo stand is organized with the femoral cannulation instruments.
      b. The second scrub nurse assists the surgeon with the femoral exposure and cannulation.
  C. Additional suture is required to close the femoral incision sites after cardiopulmonary bypass has been discontinued.
VI. Clinical Indicators for Evaluation
  A. Efficiency of preparation and institution for femoral cannulation
  B. Availability of the femoral cannulation supplies and instrumentation
  C. Staff education regarding the implementation of cardiopulmonary bypass using the femoral cannulation route
  D. Patient's response and outcome

Cardiac Surgery: Policy: Ventricular Assist Device Implantation

Cardiac surgery's policy is that the following criteria be met for the implantation of a ventricular assist device, including but not limited to

1. Perfusionist availability to monitor the VAD, 24 hours a day
2. All VAD supplies are checked prior to the start of the surgical procedure to ensure availability
3. Complete open-heart case preparation
4. The manufacturer's guidelines for implantation are followed
5. Documentation of the VAD implantation and performance
    a. Type of VAD
    b. Manufacturer of the VAD
    c. Serial and model number of the VAD
    d. Implantation sites
    e. Name of surgeon
    f. Date and time of implantation
    g. Perfusion records of cardiopulmonary bypass and VAD monitoring
    h. Patient's response to the VAD

Cardiac Surgery: Nursing Procedure: Ventricular Assist Device Implantation

Quality Outcome: Safe and effective implantation of the ventricular assist device is accomplished.

Performed by: Cardiac surgeon, cardiac anesthesiologist, perfusionist, hemodynamic monitoring specialist, circulating nurses, and scrub nurse

General Statement: The workload of the heart is decreased by diverting blood from the ventricle to an artificial pump that maintains systemic perfusion.

Equipment: Basic heart equipment, supplies, and instrumentation; VAD supplies pertinent to the type of VAD implanted

Steps:	Rationale:
1. The surgeon communicates the type of VAD to be implanted.	Facilitates the intraoperative plan of care.
2. The circulating nurse gathers the VAD supplies and opens the inflow and outflow cannulas for the scrub nurse.	The appropriate supplies are opened for the procedure.
3. The scrub nurse organizes the supplies and prepares the cannulation stitches for placement of the inflow and outflow cannulas.	The scrub nurse knows the surgery routine and the surgeon's preference for instrumentation, sutures, and equipment needed to facilitate surgical intervention.
4. The perfusionist maintains cardiopulmonary bypass and prepares the VAD. The procedure for cardiopulmonary bypass is followed.	Cardiopulmonary bypass is used for circulatory support during implantation of the VAD. The VAD maintains systemic and myocardial perfusion while promoting metabolic and hemodynamic recovery of a reversibly damaged myocardium.
5. The inflow and outflow cannulas are inserted and tunneled through to the abdominal midline. Air is removed from the circuits and the cannulas are connected.	The VAD acts as an artificial ventricle. Air is removed to prevent air embolism.

Steps:	Rationale:
6. The patient's chest may be closed or left open. If left open, the chest is covered with some sterile material sutured to the wound edges and/or covered with a plastic incise drape.	The patient will return to the operating room for removal of the device, chest closure, or heart transplantation.

7. The circulating nurse documents the following:
   a. Manufacturer
   b. Serial and model numbers
   c. Implantation site
   d. Name of surgeon implanting the device
   e. Date of implantation
   f. Patient's response to implantation
	Pertinent information is documented in the event of mechanical failure.

8. When the procedure is completed, the postoperative transfer procedure is followed.	Continuity of care is provided.
9. The perfusionist maintains documentation of the VAD performance and patient response 24 hours a day.	The perfusionist is responsible for monitoring the VAD and documenting the patient's response to therapy.

Cardiac Surgery: Standard of Care: Ventricular Assist Devices Implantation

I. Type of Ventricular Assist Devices
   A. Left ventricular assist devices (LVADs)
   B. Right ventricular assist devices (RVADs)
   C. Intra-aortic balloon pump (IABP)
   D. Extracorporeal membrane oxygenation (ECMO)
II. Indications
   A. Long-term circulatory assistance
      1. Patients with irreversible ventricular failure
         a. Bridge to cardiac transplantation
      2. Cardiopulmonary support
         a. Adult respiratory distress syndrome
III. Equipment and Supplies for Ventricular Assist Implantation
   A. Portable VAD cart
      1. Contains all LVAD and RVAD supplies
         a. VAD inflow cannulas
         b. VAD outflow cannulas
         c. VAD pumping system
      2. VAD centrifugal pump
         a. Carmeda coated circuits
      3. Supplies are checked monthly to ensure availability.
   B. Instrumentation
      1. Standard open-heart case preparation
      2. Extra vascular clamps for cannulation
IV. Special Considerations
   A. Physiologic monitoring
      1. Arterial pressure
      2. Left atrial pressure
      3. Pulmonary artery pressure
      4. CVP
      5. Cardiac output
      6. Urinary output
   B. Systemic heparinization
   C. Cardiopulmonary bypass
   D. The patient may have his or her chest left open
   E. The VAD is operated and monitored by a perfusionist 24 hours a day
   F. Blood clotting factors are available, as needed
V. Surgical Preparation
   A. Supine position

- B. The patient is prepped from the neck to knees bilaterally
- C. Cardiopulmonary bypass is instituted

VI. Left Ventricular Assist Device
 - A. The arterial cannula is inserted into the ascending aorta and tunneled out through the skin to the left of the abdominal midline.
 - B. The atrial cannula is inserted into the dome of the left atrium and tunneled out to the left of the abdominal midline.

VII. Right Ventricular Assist Device
 - A. The arterial cannula is inserted into the pulmonary artery and tunneled out to the right of the abdominal midline.
 - B. The atrial cannula is inserted into the right atrial appendage and tunneled out to the right of the abdominal midline.

VIII. Documentation
 - A. Type of VAD
 - B. Manufacturer
 - C. Serial and model numbers of the VAD
 - D. Implantation sites
 - E. Cardiopulmonary bypass perfusion record
 - F. Perfusion record of the VAD

IX. Clinical Indicators for Evaluation
 - A. Perfusionist availability
 - B. Availability of supplies needed for VAD implantation
 - C. Patient's response to VAD implantation
 - D. Team education

Cardiac Surgery: Policy: Utilization of the Intra-Aortic Balloon Pump

Cardiac surgery's policy is that an intra-aortic balloon pump with corresponding balloons be available for every cardiac surgical procedure performed if the need for counterpulsation occurs. If an intra-aortic balloon is inserted preoperatively and the patient's condition permits, a signed consent is obtained. Documentation includes but is not limited to

1. Name of surgeon inserting the balloon
2. Time of insertion
3. Site of insertion
4. Manufacturer's name and serial and model numbers of the intra-aortic balloon pump console
5. The lot number, size, and capacity of the balloon catheter
6. Color and temperature of the extremity before and after insertion of the balloon catheter
7. Peripheral pulses
8. The intra-aortic balloon pumping ratio

The manufacturer's guidelines for insertion are followed.

Intra-Aortic Balloon Pump

The intra-aortic balloon pump (IABP) is a cardiac assist device designed to increase coronary perfusion and decrease myocardial oxygen consumption using the technique of counterpulsation.

In addition to the decrease in myocardial oxygen consumption associated with the decrease in workload and the increase in myocardial oxygen supply due to the increase in coronary perfusion, secondary effects associated with counterpulsation include a decrease in heart rate, an increase in cardiac output, a decrease in systemic vascular resistance, a decrease in left ventricular end-diastolic pressure, and an increase in mean arterial pressure. With an increase in mean arterial pressure, perfusion to all organ systems will be improved.

If there is an injury to the myocardium, a series of physiologic changes occurs that results in an imbalance between the myocardial oxygen supply and demand. With cardiac failure, cardiac output fails, increasing myocardial oxygen demands. As failure progresses, a cycle develops, causing a greater imbalance between myocardial oxygen supply and demand, leading to further failure of the pumping action of the heart. The profoundly depressed left ventricle can recuperate provided the workload and accompanying myocardial oxygen needs are reduced.

Counterpulsation with the use of the IABP is achieved by placement of a 40-mm, distensible, nonthrombogenic, polyurethane balloon in the adult patient. Mounted on a vascular catheter that has multiple communications with the lumen of the balloon, this device is inserted through the femoral artery either percutaneously or via an arteriotomy. The balloon catheter is then passed retrogradely to a position in the descending thoracic aorta just distal to the left subclavian artery. The balloon is connected to the pump and inflated during diastole, which is set to occur immediately after the physiologic closure of the aortic valve, seen on the arterial wave form.

Deflation is set to occur during isovolumetric contraction by decreasing the afterload component of cardiac work. The balloon pushes oxygenated blood to the coronary arteries during diastole, increasing the blood supply to the myocardium. The balloon is timed by using the arterial wave form. The balloon can trigger at a 1–1, 1–2, 1–3, 1–4 ratio per heartbeat as needed to maintain adequate hemodynamic effects.

Indications for balloon counterpulsation include cardiogenic shock, weaning from cardiopulmonary bypass, mechanical complications of acute myocardial infarction such as papillary muscle rupture and ventricular septal defect, preinfarction and postinfarction unstable angina resistant to medial therapy, and prophylactic support for the severely ischemic myocardium during coronary angiogram or anesthesia induction. The balloon has been instrumental as a bridge to cardiac transplantation. Viable myocardium can be supported until a donor organ has been obtained.

Nursing measures specific to the patient with a balloon in place are as follows:

A. Observation for hematologic abnormalities, specifically anemia and thrombocytopenia caused by blood loss and trauma to the platelets during counterpulsation.
B. Observation for potential infections caused by indwelling catheters and invasive procedures.
C. Observation of peripheral circulation as the potential exists for femoral artery occlusion by the balloon catheter or a thrombus. Peripheral pulses are monitored frequently.
D. Immobilizing the leg with the balloon to prevent displacement and or kinking. Contraindications to the balloon's use are aortic insufficiency, dissecting aortic aneurysm, chronic end-stage heart disease, and severe vascular disease.

Cardiac Surgery: Nursing Procedure: Intraoperative Placement of the Intra-Aortic Balloon

Quality Outcome: The intra-aortic balloon is safely inserted intraoperatively to reduce left ventricular workload and increase oxygenation to the myocardium, with subsequent increase in cardiac output and systemic perfusion.

Performed by: Cardiac surgeon, perfusionist, hemodynamic monitoring specialist, circulating nurses, and scrub nurse

General Statement: The intra-aortic balloon is inserted into the descending thoracic aorta just below the left subclavian artery via the femoral artery or, if necessary, directly into the thoracic aorta. The manufacturer's guidelines for insertion are used.

Equipment: Intra-aortic balloon console, intra-aortic balloon catheters, femoral cannulation tray, arterial pressure line and transducer set, and EKG adaptor cable for the intra-aortic balloon pump

Steps:	Rationale:
1. The circulating nurse retrieves the balloon pump console, arterial pressure monitoring equipment, and intra-aortic balloon catheters.	All of the equipment necessary for balloon pump insertion is available.
2. The circulating nurse gives the scrub nurse the appropriate sized intra-aortic balloon after verification from the surgeon.	Balloons vary in size to provide 20, 30, or 40 ml of volume displacement, providing the maximum assistance without total aortic occlusion.
3. The scrub nurse assists the surgeon with the isolation of the femoral artery, passing the guidewire, dilator, and femoral sheath.	Initially, the surgeon attempts to locate the artery with a percutaneous femoral stick. If unsuccessful, a femoral cutdown is accomplished.
4. The scrub nurse removes the intra-aortic balloon from its package, leaving it in its protective tray until ready for insertion.	The protective packaging protects the balloon from potential tears during the balloon preparation.

Steps:	Rationale:

5. The scrub nurse prepares the balloon for insertion.
   a. The one-way valve is connected to the leur port.
   b. A 60-ml syringe is attached to the valve, and 30 ml of air are slowly removed, leaving the valve in place.
	Manufacturer's guidelines are followed. Vacuum is applied to the balloon to facilitate insertion.

6. After the surgeon has placed the introducer sheath into the femoral artery, the balloon catheter is removed from its protective sheath. The surgeon measures the length of balloon needed and marks it with a ligature tie.	The balloon is positioned in the descending aorta, distal to the subclavian, carotid, and innominate arteries.
7. The scrub nurse passes the arterial pressure line to the perfusionist or hemodynamic monitoring specialist standing at the balloon console.	The arterial pressure line facilitates central arterial pressure monitoring and aids in balloon pump triggering.
8. The perfusionist or hemodynamic monitoring specialist connects the pressure line to the transducer and flushes the line, removing all air. The transducer line is zero balanced.	Air is removed from the line to prevent the risk of air embolism and pressure line dampening. The transducer must be zero balanced to facilitate proper pressure monitoring.
9. The scrub nurse hands the balloon vacuum line to the perfusionist/ hemodynamic monitoring technician, who then connects it to the proper terminal of the intra-aortic balloon console.	The balloon is unwrapped after the vacuum line has been connected to the balloon pump console.
10. The perfusionist/hemodynamic monitoring specialist goes through the required safety checks and verifies the position of the balloon with the surgeon.	Counterpulsation is initiated when all of the safety checks are completed and the surgeon has verified the correct position of the balloon catheter.

Steps:	Rationale:
11. The sheath and balloon are sutured into place.	Securing the balloon in position decreases the risk of balloon dislodgement or hemorrhage.
12. After the insertion, the femoral site is observed for unusual bleeding or subcutaneous hematoma formation. The circulating nurse checks the pedal pulses, temperature, and color of the affected limb.	Complications arising from the utilization of the intra-aortic balloon are continually assessed.

13. The circulating nurse completes the required documentation, including
  a. Manufacturer, lot number, size, and volume of the balloon catheter
  b. The balloon pump console
    1. Manufacturer
    2. Serial number
    3. Model number
  c. Site of insertion
  d. Name of the surgeon inserting the balloon
  e. Balloon pump rates and ratios
  f. Intensive care documentation sheet
    1. Trigger component
    2. Balloon pump rates and ratios
    3. The patient's tolerance and response to the procedure
	Documentation of all intraoperative care is completed.

14. The intra-aortic balloon site is dressed with a dry, occlusive dressing.	The dressing prevents the risk of infection.

Steps:	Rationale:
15. The circulating nurse connects the balloon EKG cable to the EKG electrodes on the patient.	The balloon cable enables the monitoring of the patient during transport. The balloon pump is monitored by a balloon certified individual 24 hours a day, until it is no longer needed.
16. The perfusionist/hemodynamic monitoring specialist or the balloon certified staff member monitors the intra-aortic balloon to the intensive care unit. The transfer of the postoperative cardiac surgical patient is followed.	
17. When not in use, the balloon pump is kept in close proximity to the surgical suite and plugged into an electrical source.	Electricity is necessary to recharge the intra-aortic balloon pump batteries, which are used during the transport of a patient.

Standard of Care: Cardiac Surgery: Counterpulsation Using the Intra-Aortic Balloon Pump

I. Indications for Counterpulsation
   A. Cardiogenic shock or left ventricular failure
      1. Valvular disease
      2. Viral myocarditis
      3. Postoperative low output syndrome
   B. Unstable angina refractory to medical therapy
   C. In conjunction with thrombolytic therapy
   D. Management of refractory ventricular dysrhythmias
   E. Acute anterior infarction to contain the area of injury
   F. In conjunction with coronary arteriography, PTCA, and coronary stenting
      1. Prophylactic support for high-risk patients
      2. Failed angioplasty
   G. Preoperative stabilization of high-risk patients before anesthesia induction
   H. Weaning from cardiopulmonary bypass
   I. Circulatory support for cardiac transplants
   J. An adjunct to mechanical ventricular assist
II. Contraindications for Counterpulsation
   A. Irreversible brain damage
   B. Chronic and end-stage heart disease
   C. Incompetent aortic valve
   D. Dissecting aortic or thoracic aneurysms
   E. Peripheral vascular disease
III. Equipment Needed
   A. Location of equipment and supplies
      1. The balloon pump console and supplies are kept in near proximity to the cardiac surgical suite.
         a. Intra-aortic balloon pump console
         b. Intra-aortic balloon catheters
         c. Femoral cannulation tray
         d. Arterial pressure line and transducer
         e. EKG cable adaptor for the balloon pump console
IV. Insertion Site
   A. Femoral artery
      1. Percutaneous
      2. Femoral artery cutdown

- B. Aorta
  1. Directly into the thoracic aorta
- C. The balloon catheter is inserted according to the manufacturer's guidelines.
- D. The balloon catheter is secured in place with suture material after the correct position of the catheter has been confirmed.
  1. An x-ray may be taken to confirm the correct position of the balloon.

V. Intra-Aortic Balloon Pump Monitoring
- A. Personnel monitoring balloon pump function
  1. Surgeon
  2. Perfusionist
  3. Hemodynamic monitoring specialist
  4. Licensed personnel that have been trained in counterpulsation techniques
     a. Intra-aortic balloon class
     b. Proctored on a specified number of cases
     c. Documented skills checklist

VI. Circulating Nurse's Responsibilities
- A. Assistance with retrieving the balloon pump console and the balloon catheters
- B. Opening the balloon catheter on the sterile field for the scrub nurse/tech
- C. Perioperative nursing assessment before and after the balloon insertion
- D. Complete documentation of the procedure and the patient's response

VII. Scrub Nurse/Tech Responsibilities
- A. Educated in the sequence of events for insertion of the balloon
  1. How the balloon works
  2. Preparation of the balloon
  3. Preparation of the arterial pressure line
  4. Femoral cannulation instruments available should a cutdown become necessary
  5. Availability of the appropriate suture

VIII. Perioperative Nursing Assessments
- A. Observation anteriorly and posteriorly for blood hematoma
- B. Presence of peripheral pulses
  1. Strength
  2. Color and warmth of the limb
- C. Observation of augmentation
  1. Awareness of the trigger component
     a. Arterial blood pressure
     b. Electrocardiogram

IX. Documentation
   A. Name of the surgeon inserting the balloon
   B. Time of insertion
   C. Site of insertion
   D. Manufacturer's name and serial and model numbers of the intra-aortic balloon pump console
   E. The lot number, size, and capacity of the balloon catheter
   F. Color and temperature of the extremity before and after insertion of the balloon catheter
   G. Peripheral pulses
   H. The intra-aortic balloon pumping ratio
X. Maintenance of the Intra-Aortic Balloon Pump Console
   A. A team member is assigned to ensure that the balloon pump is available and plugged into an electrical outlet to keep the battery charged.
   B. Routine maintenance is performed according to hospital policy.
XI. Transfer of the Patient with an Intra-Aortic Balloon
   A. Balloon EKG cables are connected to the EKG leads on the patient.
   B. The intra-aortic balloon pump is capable of monitoring hemodynamic parameters.
      1. Monitors the heart rate and rhythm
      2. Monitors the arterial blood pressure
         a. Actual
         b. Augmented
      3. Requires additional assistance to safely transport the patient to the unit
      4. Counterpulsation pumping ratios and triggering information are documented on the intensive care documentation sheet.
XII. Clinical Indicators for Evaluation
   A. Balloon pump availability and accessibility
   B. Complications associated with insertion of the intra-aortic balloon
   C. Team's response for insertion of the balloon
      1. Education of team members
         a. Skills checklist
   D. Patient's response to counterpulsation therapy

Cardiac Surgery: Policy: Pacing of the Cardiac Surgical Patient

Cardiac surgery's policy is that supplies and equipment are available for temporary or permanent pacing during every cardiac surgical procedure if the need arises to treat conduction disturbances affecting the rate or rhythm of the contracting heart.

Cardiac Surgery: Nursing Procedure: Intraoperative Placement of Temporary Pacing Electrodes

Quality Outcome: Artificial pacing is instituted to re-establish a rhythm conducive to an adequate cardiac output.

Performed by: Cardiac surgeon, cardiac anesthesiologist, circulating nurse, and scrub nurse

General Statement: The selection of the pacing system and electrode placement is dependent on the specific pacing requirements of the individual patient.

Equipment: Pulse generator, alligator clips, atrial pacing electrodes, ventricular pacing electrodes, and pacing cables

Steps:	Rationale:
1. The scrub nurse has alligator clips and atrial and ventricular cables opened on her sterile field for every open-heart procedure. Pacing electrode wires are in the surgical suite if needed.	Temporary pacing equipment is available throughout the duration of the case if pacing becomes necessary.
2. The hemodynamic monitoring specialist checks the pulse generator before the start of the procedure.	A pulse generator is available and has been checked to ensure that the battery is viable.
3. In an emergency, when pacing is required, the alligator clips are used while the temporary wires are being placed.	Alligator clips can be attached directly to the myocardium and connected to a pulse generator, providing temporary pacing immediately.
4. The scrub nurse anticipates the need for temporary pacing and prepares the pacing wires according to the type of pacing required.	The scrub nurse is constantly aware of the EKG changes that may necessitate a change in the normal routine of the procedure.
5. The surgeon requests the type of pacing required.	Pacing may include atrial, ventricular, or A–V sequential dependent on the need of the patient.

Steps:	Rationale:
6. The scrub nurse prepares the electrode wires used for ventricular pacing by loading the curved needle on the electrode wire on a needle holder. A small wire scissor is available to remove the curved needle after the correct placement of the electrode wire. The straight needles on the other end of the electrodes are tunneled out through the skin on the left side of the chest wall and are attached to the ventricular pacing cable, which is connected to the pulse generator. The wires are secured to the chest wall with a suture.	Two myocardial leads are attached to the left ventricle for ventricular pacing. After the lead has been attached, the curved needle is removed, leaving the electrode attached to the ventricular wall. The pulse generator provides the electrical current needed to pace the heart. The ventricular pacing cable helps keep the electrode wires from coming in contact with each other, causing a short in the system. The ventricular cable is labeled "ventricular" for quick and easy identification of the electrodes postoperatively. The wires are secured with a suture to the skin to prevent the accidental dislodgement of the pacing wires.
7. The anesthesiologist sets the rate and demand according to the surgeon's request and the patient's response to therapy.	A rhythm conducive to maintain an adequate cardiac output is established with the help of the temporary pacemaker.
8. The scrub nurse prepares the electrode wires providing temporary pacing immediately.	The atrial wires are secured on the right atrium. The pulse generator provides the electrical current needed to pace the heart. The atrial pacing cable helps keep the electrode wires from coming in contact with each other, causing a short in the system. The atrial cable is labeled "atrial" to provide quick and easy identification of the electrodes postoperatively. The wires are secured in place with a suture to prevent the accidental dislodgement of the wires.

Steps:	Rationale:
9. The anesthesiologist sets the rate and demand according to the surgeon's request and the patient's response to therapy.	A rhythm conducive to maintain an adequate cardiac output is established with the help of the temporary pacemaker.
10. The circulating nurse documents the placement and location of the temporary pacing wires on the surgical record and the intensive care documentation sheet.	Intraoperative care is recorded. Continuity of care is provided by a verbal or written report to the intensive care unit.

Cardiac Surgery: Nursing Procedure: Insertion of a Permanent Pacemaker

Quality Outcome: Permanent pacing of the myocardium is accomplished to establish a rhythm conducive to an adequate cardiac output.

Performed by: Cardiac surgeon, cardiac anesthesiologist, circulating nurse, and scrub nurse

General Statement: A permanent pacemaker, consisting of a generator and electrodes, initiates atrial, ventricular, or both types of contractions to treat conduction disturbances affecting the rate or rhythm of the contracting heart.

Equipment: Pulse generator, pacing analyzer, alligator clips, sterile pacemaker, pacing electrodes, defibrillator, and emergency drugs

Steps:	Rationale:
1. The surgeon communicates to the team the type of anesthesia to be used, surgical approach, and the type of permanent pacemaker that is to be used.	The pacemaker may be inserted under local, general, or monitored anesthesia care. All supplies are organized and checked before the beginning of the case.
2. The room is prepared with the following equipment but not limited to a. Defibrillator b. Emergency drugs c. Surgery table that accommodates a C-arm x-ray machine d. Lead aprons	Dysrhythmias can occur during catheter insertion. Fluoroscopy is needed to visualize the correct placement of the transvenous pacing leads. The hospital's policy regarding the use of x-rays and protective apparel is followed.
3. The patient is placed in a supine position and connected to noninvasive monitoring equipment, including but not limited to a. Blood pressure monitor b. EKG monitor c. Pulse oximeter	Continuous monitoring of the patient's hemodynamics is essential.

Steps:	Rationale:
4. The circulating nurse preps the surgical sites for electrode and generator insertion. The subclavian region is prepped if the surgeon is inserting endocardial pacing electrodes and the sub-xiphoid area is prepped if the surgeon is placing epicardial leads. A pocket is created for the pacemaker generator.	Several incision sites are necessary for the pacemaker and electrode insertion. The surgical sites are prepped to decrease microorganisms on the skin, reducing the risk of infection.
5. The scrub nurse prepares the instrumentation that is appropriate for the surgical approach. Alligator clips are available, if needed, before insertion of the electrodes. When the leads are positioned, they are attached to an external pacemaker or a pacing analyzer.	The scrub nurse knows the routine for the procedure and the surgeon's preference for sutures used. The leads are tested to ensure adequate capture.
6. The pocket is created for the generator. A subcutaneous tunnel is formed with a blunt instrument.	The electrodes are tunneled through the subcutaneous tissue and are connected to the generator.
7. The circulating nurse documents the manufacturer and serial and model numbers, rate and site of pacing electrode and generator, and implantation date and time and completes the patient's identification card and pacemaker registration.	Intraoperative care is documented. Patients with a pacemaker require adequate follow-up to prevent possible complications.

Cardiac Surgery: Nursing Procedure: Insertion of a Permanent Pacemaker

Standard of Care: Cardiac Surgery: Pacemakers

I. Indications for a Pacemaker
   A. Treatment of dysrhythmias
      1. Bradycardias
      2. Complete heart block
      3. Tachyarrhythmias
II. Selection of the Pacemaker System
   A. Dependent on the specific needs of the patient
      1. Temporary
         a. Used to treat transient forms of heart block and dysrhythmias that occasionally occur during cardiac surgery
         b. Used before implantation of a permanent pacemaker
      2. Permanent
         a. Complete heart block
      3. Unipolar or bipolar
III. Pulse Generators
   A. Classified into three groups
      1. Fixed rate
      2. Ventricular demand
      3. Physiologic
IV. Methods of Electrode Placement
   A. Transvenous
   B. Epicardial
   C. Subxiphoid
V. Placement of Electrode Leads
   A. Endocardial
      1. Inserted transvenously
   B. Epicardial
      1. Attached to the heart muscle under direct vision
VI. Methods of Electrode Placement
   A. Transvenous
   B. Epicardial
   C. Subxiphoid
VII. Special Equipment
   A. Temporary pacing
      1. Pacing electrodes
         a. Atrial
         b. Ventricular
      2. Pacing cables

          3. Pulse generator
          4. Sutures for securing the wires
     B. Permanent
          1. Pacing electrodes
          2. Pacing cables
          3. Alligator clips
          4. Pulse generator
          5. Sterile pacemaker
          6. Pacing analyzer

VIII. Special Considerations
     A. Supine position
     B. Continuous electrocardiographic monitoring
     C. Defibrillator
     D. Emergency drugs are available.
     E. Fluoroscopy required
          a. Via the transvenous route
     F. Electrocautery units are used with caution after the generator placement.

IX. Documentation
     A. Temporary pacing
          1. Location of wires
               a. Atrial
               b. Ventricular
               c. Atrial–ventricular
          2. Rate
     B. Permanent pacing
          1. Manufacturer
               a. Serial and model numbers of the pacemaker and electrodes
               b. Rate
               c. Route of implantation of the pacing wires
               d. Date and time of insertion
               e. Patient registration and identification cards

X. Clinical Indicators for Evaluation
     A. Availability of pacing systems
     B. Staff education
     C. Patient response to therapy
     D. Complete documentation

Cardiac Surgery: Policy: Implantation of the Automatic Internal Cardioverter Defibrillator

Cardiac surgery's policy is that the following criteria be met when implanting an automatic internal cardioverter defibrillator, including but not limited to

1. The surgical approach is verified.
2. The manufacturer's guidelines for implantation are followed.
3. A defibrillator is available at all times.
4. Equipment needed for internal defibrillation is available.
5. Antidysrhythmic drugs are readily available.
6. Appropriate documentation is completed.
    a. Manufacturer's name
    b. Model and serial number of the AICD
    c. Implantation sites for the electrodes and the defibrillator generator
    d. Specific parameters used to determine the dysrhythmia
    e. Patient registration and identification cards

Cardiac Surgery: Nursing Procedure: Implantation of the Automatic Internal Cardioverter Defibrillator

Quality Outcome: Safe and effective implantation of the AICD is accomplished.
Performed by: Cardiac surgeon, circulating nurse, and scrub nurse
General Statement: Sensing electrodes are positioned on the epicardium to monitor changes in the heart rate and cycle length waveform, delivering a synchronized countershock if necessary.
Equipment: Defibrillator, AICD system, internal paddles and cords, and antidysrhythmic drugs

Steps:	Rationale:
1. The circulating nurse verifies the correct surgical approach.	Facilitates the perioperative plan of care.
2. The patient is positioned and prepped according to the surgical approach used.	Two incision sites are required. One is for the placement of the epicardial wires; the other is for the defibrillator generator.
3. The internal paddles from the sterile field are connected to the defibrillator. External defibrillating pads may be used for this procedure.	Countershock may become necessary at any time during the surgical procedure. External defibrillating pads facilitate defibrillation without disrupting the integrity of the sterile field after the surgical incision has been made.
4. The scrub nurse assists the surgeon as needed.	The scrub nurse knows the surgery routine and the surgeon's preference for instrumentation, sutures, and equipment.
5. The circulating nurse assists the anesthesiologist.	Emergency support of the patient is facilitated with experienced teamwork involvement.

Steps:	Rationale:
6. The circulating nurse has the defibrillator ready at all times.	Dysrhythmia induction and termination are performed in two stages. The first stage is before the device-to-lead connection is made. The second stage is after the device-to-lead connection has occurred to ensure the device reliability of detection and countershock delivery.

7. Documentation of the procedure includes but is not limited to
   a. Name, model number, and serial number of the AICD
   b. Site of implantation
   c. Parameter settings for therapy
      1. Heart rate
      2. Density function
   d. Patient's registration card
	Facilitates long-term follow-up care and research.

Cardiac Surgery: Standard of Care: Implantation of an Automatic Internal Cardioverter Defibrillator

I. Indications for an Automatic Internal Cardioverter Defibrillator
   A. Sudden cardiac death
   B. Recurrent ventricular dysrhythmias despite conventional antidysrhythmic drug therapy
      1. Ventricular tachycardia
      2. Ventricular fibrillation
II. Surgical Positioning
   A. Median sternotomy
   B. Left lateral thoracotomy
   C. Subxiphoid
   D. Subcostal implantation
III. Perioperative Planning
   A. Surgical approach
   B. Appropriate instrumentation and supplies
   C. Appropriate equipment
IV. Equipment
   A. Automatic internal cardioverter defibrillator system (AICD)
      1. Pulse generator
      2. Two electrodes with the corresponding leads
   B. Defibrillator
V. Instrumentation and Supplies
   A. Instruments appropriate for the surgical approach used
   B. Appropriate suture material
   C. Internal defibrillator paddles
   D. Antidysrhythmic drugs
   E. Temporary pacing leads and pulse generator
VI. Documentation
   A. Manufacturer's name
   B. Model and serial numbers of the AICD
   C. Implantation sites of the electrodes and the defibrillator generator
   D. Specific patient parameters used to determine a dysrhythmia:
      1. The heart rate of the patient's that overrides the AICD device causing initiation of countershock therapy
      2. Density function of the device
         a. Measurement based on the shape of the electrocardiogram with a relative time at an isolated baseline

    E. Patient registration and identification cards
VII. Clinical Indicators for Evaluation
    A. The patient's response to therapy
    B. Complications encountered
    C. Availability of supplies and instrumentation
    D. Staff education

Cardiac Surgery: Policy: Reimplementation of Cardiopulmonary Bypass

Cardiac surgery's policy is that the following criteria be followed to facilitate the reinstitution of cardiopulmonary bypass safely, quickly, and efficiently to promote cardiac life support. Criteria include but are not limited to the following:

1. The perfusionist remains in the surgery department until the patient has been safely transferred to the intensive care unit.
2. Backup perfusion supplies are stored in the surgical suite for quick and easy accessibility.
3. The extracorporeal circuits remain on the sterile field until the sternum has been reapproximated with surgical wire.
4. The reservoir on the oxygenator is not depleted beyond the level of fluid that would permit immediate reinstitution of bypass until specific and confirmed approval of the surgeon has been given.
5. Team role responsibilities are discussed, with guidelines developed for the intraoperative plan of care.

Cardiac Surgery: Nursing Procedure: Reimplementation of Cardiopulmonary Bypass

Quality Outcome: Cardiopulmonary bypass is reestablished quickly, efficiently, and effectively to promote cardiac life support until other definitive measures can be instituted, according to the patient's immediate clinical status.

Performed by: Cardiac surgeon, cardiac anesthesiologist, perfusionist, circulating nurses, hemodynamic monitoring specialist, and scrub nurse

General Statement: The entire cardiac team is constantly aware of the progression of the case and the clinical status of the patient to be able to prioritize actions in an emergency situation.

Equipment: Heart–lung machine; extracorporeal circuit; perfusion cannulas, venous and arterial; cannulation stitches and ligature ties; intra-aortic balloon pump and catheters; alligator clips and pacemaker generator; and stat lab equipment

Steps:	Rationale:
1. The team is aware of the case progression and the patient's hemodynamic status throughout the intraoperative procedure.	The intraoperative plan of care is revised, as needed, to meet the changing hemodynamic status of the patient.
2. ACLS is initiated by the team as the patient's clinical status warrants and until cardiopulmonary bypass can be reinstituted.	Actions are prioritized and directed at maintaining adequate oxygenation and cardiac output conducive with life.

Steps:	Rationale:

3. The perfusionist assesses the status of the extracorporeal circuit and prioritizes actions accordingly, coordinating efforts with the scrub nurse and the surgeon.
   a. Circuits that remain on the sterile field and are not emptied do not need to be re-primed unless there is air in the system.
   b. Empty circuits remaining on the sterile field need to be re-primed prior to cannulation. A 3/8" × 1/2" straight connector is given to the scrub nurse to join the arterial and venous circuits together to permit the perfusionist to prime the circuits.
   c. If the extracorporeal circuits have been discarded, new circuits are opened, secured to the surgical drapes, and primed. After the arterial–venous circuit has been primed, the perfusionist tells the scrub nurse to divide the circuit.
	The perfusionist is responsible for the extracorporeal circuits and ensures that they are accurately prepared for cardiopulmonary bypass. Air in the circuits may cause air embolism. The scrub nurse knows the diameters of the different extracorporeal circuits to facilitate all necessary circuit connections.
	
	Actions are prioritized to facilitate cardiopulmonary bypass.
	
	All air is removed from the circuit.
	
	The arterial–venous circuit is divided to provide two separate circuits, a venous return circuit and an arterial circuit.

4. The circulating nurse calls for extra assistance if needed. The circulating nurse facilitates the reimplementation of cardiopulmonary bypass by opening supplies and sutures needed by the scrub nurse.	Extra assistance may be necessary to organize supplies and coordinate the ACLS efforts. The circulating nurse is aware of the supplies and sutures needed by the scrub nurse.

Steps:	Rationale:
5. The scrub nurse's priorities are to ensure that the perfusion catheters are available, cannulation stitches are ready, the extracorporeal table circuits are ready to connect to the perfusion catheters, and heparin is available if the patient has been reversed with protamine.	Arterial and venous cannulation is done before cardiopulmonary bypass can be initiated. It is the responsibility of the scrub nurse to ensure that the extracorporeal table circuit, perfusion cannulas, and cannulation stitches are prepared. Systemic anticoagulation is necessary to prevent clot formation within the extracorporeal circuit during cardiopulmonary bypass.
6. The second circulator assists the first circulator with gathering and opening the appropriate supplies and then scrubs to assist the first scrub nurse.	Effective teamwork is essential as needed to prevent or diminish catastrophic events intraoperatively. Time is life for cardiac surgery patients.
7. After cardiopulmonary bypass has been reinstituted, the cardiopulmonary bypass procedure is followed.	The perfusionist implements cardiopulmonary bypass under the direction and supervision of the cardiac surgeon.
8. The circulating nurse has the intraaortic balloon pump and balloon catheters available should they be required to wean the patient successfully from cardiopulmonary bypass.	Counterpulsation therapy may be instituted to augment the patient's cardiac output, permitting separation from cardiopulmonary bypass.
9. Documentation is continued on the following records: a. Operative report b. Anesthesia record c. Perfusion record d. Fluid flow sheet e. Variance report sheet f. Intensive care documentation sheet	All intraoperative care is documented.

Standard of Care: Cardiac Surgery: Reimplementation of Cardiopulmonary Bypass

I. Main Objectives
   A. Advanced cardiac life support
   B. Quick and efficient implementation of extracorporeal circulation
   C. Establishment of team priorities for the care executed to meet the needs of the patient
II. Special Considerations
   A. The integrity of the sterile field is not disturbed until the patient has been safely transferred to the intensive care unit.
   B. The extracorporeal table circuits remain on the surgical field until the patient is hemodynamically stable, and the mediastinum has been re-approximated with sternal wire.
   C. Backup perfusion supplies are immediately available in the surgical suite.
      1. Perfusion cannulas
         a. Aortic and femoral arterial cannulas
         b. Atrial and femoral venous cannulas
      2. Priming fluids
      3. Heparin supply
      4. The extracorporeal circuit for the heart–lung machine and the surgical field
   D. A circulating nurse remains in the surgery suite at all times.
   E. The team is constantly aware of the progression of the case, the status of extracorporeal circulation using cardiopulmonary bypass, and the changes in the patient's hemodynamics.
III. Special Considerations for the Perfusionist
   A. The perfusionist remains in the surgery department until the patient has been safely transferred to the intensive care unit.
   B. The perfusionist is available for all mediastinal re-exploration procedures within the first 24 hours postoperatively.
   C. The extracorporeal circuits are organized for quick, safe, and effective assembly.
IV. Special Considerations for the Scrub Nurse/Tech
   A. The scrub nurse/tech retains an additional set of cannulation suture on the sterile field at all times.
   B. The instruments and supplies are kept organized throughout the entire procedure.

C. The scrub nurse/tech is aware of the administration of heparin, the reversal of heparin with protamine, and the patient's response.
D. The scrub nurse/tech is aware of the status of the extracorporeal circuit at all times.
   1. Actions are prioritized according to the following criteria:
      a. If and when systemic heparinization or protamine reversal has occurred
         1. Protamine, if being administered, is discontinued.
         2. If protamine reversal has been completed, the initial heparin dose is redrawn and administered before cardiopulmonary bypass.
   2. If the arterial or venous cannulas are removed, but the extracorporeal circuit remains on the field
      a. The surgeon may need to reheparinize depending on the status of the protamine administration.
      b. Arterial and/or venous cannulation stitches are prepared.
      c. Re-priming of the extracorporeal arterial–venous loop on the table circuit
         1. A 1/20 × 3/80 straight connector is opened, connected to the arterial cannula if not using a cannula with a built-in connector, and connected to the venous tubing to prime the circuit with fluid, clearing it of all air.
   3. If the extracorporeal circuit has been removed from the sterile field and discarded:
      a. Administration of heparin by the surgeon or anesthesiologist
      b. Preparation and assistance with placement of the cannulation stitches
      c. The extracorporeal table circuits are opened for use on the sterile field and secured to the surgical drapes, handing the ends of the circuit to the perfusionist.
      d. The table circuit is connected to the heart–lung machine and is primed with fluid.
      e. At the signal from the perfusionist, the arterial–venous loop is divided, creating a venous and arterial side to the circuits.
      f. The arterial and venous perfusion cannulas are ready for placement.
V. Special Considerations for the Circulating Nurse
   A. Heparin is available to give to the scrub nurse/tech.
   B. The circulating nurse is familiar with the perfusion supplies, cannulas, and their locations.
      1. The circulating nurse anticipates needs and has the appropriate supplies available.

        2. Additional sutures are available and added to the needle count.
    C. The second circulating nurse scrubs to assist the first scrub nurse prepare the extracorporeal circuit, if needed.
    D. The intensive care unit is notified that cardiopulmonary bypass has been re-established.
    E. After cardiopulmonary bypass has been initiated, the appropriate communication is relayed to the family.
    F. The circulating nurse has the intra-aortic balloon pump and balloon catheters in the surgical suite.
VI. Documentation
    A. Variance report sheet
    B. Perfusion record
    C. Operative report
    D. Anesthesia report
    E. Fluid documentation sheet
    F. Intensive care documentation sheet
VII. Clinical Indicators for Evaluation
    A. Timeliness and effectiveness of team response for reestablishing cardiopulmonary bypass
    B. The effectiveness of advanced cardiac life support
    C. Availability of supplies
    D. The patient's response to the therapy instituted

Cardiac Surgery: Policy: Re-Exploration of the Mediastinum for Hemorrhage

Cardiac surgery's policy is that the entire cardiac surgical team be present to facilitate and expedite the surgical process to control postoperative hemorrhage when returning a cardiac surgical patient less than 24 hours postoperatively to surgery. The team includes but is not limited to

1. Cardiac surgeon
2. Cardiac anesthesiologist
3. Perfusionist
4. Hemodynamic monitoring specialist
5. Circulating nurses
6. Scrub nurse

Emergency equipment along with supplies and equipment needed for cardiopulmonary bypass is available if extracorporeal circulation should become necessary to control postoperative hemorrhage.

Cardiac Surgery: Nursing Procedure: Re-Exploration of the Mediastinum for Hemorrhage

Quality Outcome: Postoperative hemorrhage is controlled with maintenance of the patient's hemodynamic status through the coordinated efforts of the cardiac surgical team to expedite the return to surgery, facilitate surgical intervention, and replace lost, circulating blood volume.

Performed by: Cardiac surgeon, cardiac anesthesiologist, perfusionist, hemodynamic monitoring specialist, circulating nurses, and scrub nurse

General Statement: Patients requiring re-exploration of the mediastinum may present in a stable or very unstable condition. Priorities are established for care delivered to accomplish optimal patient outcomes.

Equipment: Basic heart tray of instruments, major custom pack of supplies, internal defibrillating cords and paddles, alligator clips, fibrillator box or off-pump supplies, perfusion supplies available but not opened, cannulation suture/ligature ties, pledgets, sternal wire, fascia and skin suture, cardiovascular needles if a CABG case, and autotransfusion unit and aspiration circuit

Steps:	Rationale:
1. The cardiac manager coordinates the mobilization of the cardiac team, communicating the sense of urgency and condition of the patient. The type of surgery the patient has undergone is communicated to the team.	The cardiac manager is responsible for contacting the cardiac team. Team communication facilitates case preparation and enables the team to plan the methods of perioperative patient care. A brief report of the type of surgical procedure the patient has previously undergone facilitates the organization of the correct supplies, instrumentation, and equipment.
2. The circulating nurse checks to ensure that all cardiac equipment is available and plugged in to the appropriate power sources. Wall suction is available to connect to the pleural drainage canister after transfer has been made to the surgical suite.	All cardiac surgical equipment and emergency equipment is ready before transport. The pleural drainage unit must be connected to suction until the mediastinum is opened to prevent tamponade.

Steps:	Rationale:
3. The scrub nurse gathers and opens the appropriate supplies and suture.	The scrub nurse knows the surgeon's routine and suture preference and tries to anticipate the needs of the patient and the surgeon.
4. The perfusionist is available to prepare the heart–lung machine if needed and to assist with the transport of the patient to surgery and with room preparation to facilitate surgical intervention.	Cardiopulmonary bypass may be necessary to repair or correct the hemorrhagic process.
5. The fibrillator box, off-pump supplies, and alligator clips are available.	The fibrillator causes fibrillation, enabling the surgeon to accomplish a quick repair without the need to arrest the heart totally with cardioplegia. The off-pump supplies may be utilized to stabilize a beating heart while the surgeon places stitches around a bleeding anastomosis without instituting CPB as long as the patient is hemodynamically stable.
6. The procedure for the transfer of the unstable patient to surgery is followed.	All attempts are made to expedite surgical intervention.
7. The mediastinal drainage unit is connected to suction upon arrival in the surgical suite. If a continuous autotransfusion pleural drainage unit is used, the blood collected in the reservoir is returned to the patient.	Continuous suction is applied to the unit until the mediastinum is opened to prevent cardiac tamponade. The pleural autotransfusion unit permits replacement of blood loss with the patient's own blood.
8. Bank blood is retrieved. The circulating nurse keeps a certain number of units ahead of the specific demand of the patient.	Assures blood availability, as the need for blood transfusion arises to maintain the patient's hemodynamic stability.

Steps:	Rationale:
9. The patient is placed in a supine position. Noninvasive monitors are placed. Arms are padded and tucked at the patient's sides, and the dispersive electrode pad is positioned. The sternal dressings are removed, and the circulating nurse preps from the chin to the knees bilaterally.	The surgical position is dependent on optimal exposure to the operative site and patient safety. The femoral arteries are exposed for surgical access, if needed, for intra-aortic balloon placement.

10. The scrub nurse completes the draping procedure for a mediastinal procedure, including but not limited to
  a. Four towels positioned around the original surgical incision
  b. Four towel clips or a plastic incise drape to keep the towels in place
  c. A drape extending over the legs
  d. A drape extending over the arms and head
  e. A laparotomy sheet
	Draping creates a sterile barrier and isolates the area of exposure.

11. The circulating nurse and the hemodynamic monitoring specialist connect the equipment from the field, including but not limited to
  a. Cautery
  b. Autotransfusion aspirating line
  c. Internal defibrillating paddles
	Priority of needs is established to facilitate surgical intervention.

Steps:	Rationale:
12. The scrub nurse is ready with the instruments needed to re-explore the mediastinum. Instruments needed first are a. Staple remover, if skin staples present b. Knife c. Wire cutter d. Heavy needle holder e. Sponges f. Sternal retractor g. Suction h. Cautery The sternal wires must be removed before the mediastinum can be re-explored.	The scrub nurse prioritizes and anticipates the needs of the patient and surgeon to facilitate surgical intervention.
13. Physiological monitoring intraoperatively is completed by the perfusionist or hemodynamic monitoring specialist, including but not limited to a. Arterial blood gases b. Electrolytes c. Glucose, if warranted d. Hematocrit and hemoglobin e. Heparin protamine titrations f. Acid–base balances	The stat lab provides the capability to perform the lab tests quickly and efficiently to enable the team to take the appropriate action.
14. If cardiopulmonary bypass becomes necessary, the guidelines for implementation of extracorporeal circulation are followed.	Cardiopulmonary bypass may be necessary to control the mediastinal hemorrhage and provide hemodynamic stability for the critical cardiac patient.
15. After completion of the surgical procedure and stabilization of the patient's hemodynamics, the patient is transferred to the intensive care unit.	The procedure for postoperative patient transfer is followed.

Cardiac Surgery: Standard of Care: Re-Exploration of the Mediastinum for Hemorrhage

I. Main Objectives
   A. Control of hemorrhage
      1. The patient's mediastinum may be opened in the unit with control of hemorrhage by manual pressure and/or occlusive clamping at the site of bleeding.
   B. Replacement of lost blood volume
      1. Blood/blood products
      2. Plasma
      3. Fluids
   C. Maintain hemodynamic stability
      1. Cardiac supportive drugs
   D. Expedite the return to surgery
      1. The entire cardiac team is notified and responds within 30 minutes.

II. Surgical Preparation
   A. The emergency re-exploration case cart of supplies, opened and organized by the scrub nurse.
      1. Major custom pack of general surgical supplies
      2. Perfusion supplies are available, but not opened, unless needed.
      3. Suture
          a. Cannulation suture/ligature ties
          b. Pledgets
          c. Sternal wire
          d. Cardiovascular needles, if a CABG case
          e. Fascia and skin suture
   B. Instrumentation; cardiopulmonary bypass may become necessary to control hemorrhage.
      1. Basic cardiac instruments
      2. A set of internal defibrillating paddles
      3. Alligator clips
   C. The autotransfusion machine is prepared, and the aspiration system is opened on the field.
   D. All cardiac standard equipment is plugged into electrical outlets and ready to use, as needed.
   E. A fibrillator box is available.
   F. Off-pump supplies are available
   G. Wall suction is available to connect to the pleural drainage unit upon transfer of the patient to surgery.

    H. The transport monitor is taken to the unit to assist with hemodynamic monitoring during the transfer.
    I. Bank blood is retrieved from the blood bank.
     1. The blood warmer is available.
     2. Pressure bags are available to pump the blood to the patient.
    J. Hemostatic agents are available.
     1. Thrombin and gelfoam
     2. Surgicele
     3. Avitene
     4. Cryoglue
     5. Flowseal
 III. Transfer of the Patient to Surgery
    A. The unstable patient transfer procedure is used.
 IV. Perioperative Priorities
    A. Positioning
     1. Supine, arms tucked at the sides
    B. Continuous hemodynamic monitoring
     1. The monitoring lines from the transport monitor are transferred to the cardiac monitor in the surgical suite.
    C. The pleural drainage unit is connected to continuous suction.
     1. The blood collected in the pleural drainage unit is reinfused to the patient.
    D. The dispersive electrode pad is positioned.
    E. The sternal dressings are removed, and the patient is prepped from the jaw to the thighs.
    F. The surgeons are scrubbed.
    G. All equipment from the field is connected and working.
     1. Cautery
     2. Autotransfusion aspiration line
     3. Internal defibrillating cords
    H. Re-entry into the mediastinum
     1. Knife blade
     2. Wire cutter
     3. Heavy needle holder
     4. Sternal retractor
     5. Sponges
 V. Perioperative Documentation
    A. Surgical operative record
    B. Fluid documentation sheet
    C. Intensive care unit documentation sheet
    D. Anesthesia record
    E. Variance report sheet

        F. Perfusion record, if warranted
VI. Patient Transport to the Intensive Care Unit
        A. The procedure for postoperative patient transport is followed.
VII. Quality Indicators for Evaluation of Care Rendered
        A. Team response time
            1. Efficiency and timeliness in transport of the patient to surgery
        B. Amount of re-exploration procedures
            1. Within 24 hours postoperatively
            2. After 24 hours postoperatively
        C. Patient outcome
            1. Hemorrhage controlled
            2. Infection rate
            3. Significant complications relating to the procedure
            4. Number of intraoperative mortalities relating to re-exploration

Cardiac Surgery: Policy: Intraoperative Mortality

Cardiac surgery's policy is that any patient who expires in the surgical suite receives appropriate and respectful care after death with strict guidelines followed to comply with state and local regulations. The healthcare team offers support for the family, as needed.

Cardiac Surgery: Nursing Procedure: Coping with Intraoperative Mortality

Quality Outcome: All patients who expire in the surgical suite will receive appropriate and respectful care after death.

Performed by: Surgeon, circulating nurse, scrub nurse, and hemodynamic monitoring nurse

General Statement: This procedure should always be in compliance with the medical examiner's guidelines.

Equipment: Morgue pack, disposition of body form, autopsy form, and medical examiner's case criteria

Steps:	Rationale:
1. The surgeon pronounces the patient to be dead and documents the appropriate information in the progress notes. The family/next of kin is notified.	It is the surgeon's responsibility to pronounce the expiration of the patient and to inform the family or next of kin.
2. The circulating nurse notifies the cardiac manager or the supervisor designee.	The nurse manager is the liaison between the healthcare team and the family to coordinate the appropriate consents for the disposition of the body and personal effects.
3. The circulating nurse notifies the medical examiner's office of the death. The body is not moved, and lines remain intact, until permission is granted from the medical examiner's office.	All intraoperative deaths are reported to the medical examiner.
4. The nurse manager obtains the mortuary release form, autopsy form, if applicable, and disposition of body form.	The family of the deceased is assisted with the arrangements for the disposition of the body.

Steps:	Rationale:
5. The circulating nurse obtains a morgue pack.	The morgue pack contains the items necessary to deliver the postmortem care.
6. After permission to implement postmortem care has been received from the medical examiner's office, all lines and tubes are removed from the body. The body is cleaned and remains in a supine position, with the arms at the sides.	Postmortem care is carried out.
7. The nurse manager discusses with the family the desire for viewing the body. If it is the family's desire to view the body, the circulating nurse moves the body to a clean, private area in the surgery department. The team provides support to the family as needed.	The family is given time to view the body and grieve.
8. When family visitation is completed, the body is tagged for proper identification and placed in a body bag. The circulating nurse ensures that the appropriate paperwork accompanies the patient. Transporters take the body to the morgue.	The body is properly identified and in the morgue within 2 hours after death.

Steps:

9. The circulating nurse completes the appropriate documentation, including but not limited to
   a. Surgical record
   b. Completed nursing notes
      1. Sequence of events
      2. Time of death
      3. Name of surgeon pronouncing the patient
      4. Name of the medical examiner giving permission to proceed with the postmortem care
      5. Completion of a CPR record, if indicated
      6. Variance report
      7. Name of transporters delivering the body to the morgue
      8. Time the body is transported to the morgue

10. The staff is given time to express its feelings about the death. Acknowledgment of efforts and limitations is shared.

Rationale:

All documentation is completed and in medical records within 2 hours of death.

The healthcare team's concept of care is geared toward survival. The team expects the patient to leave the operating room alive. Feelings of helplessness, frustration, guilt, and anger are common feelings.

Standard of Care: Cardiac Surgery: Intraoperative Mortality

I. Implementation of the Postmortem Process
   A. Pronouncement of death
      1. Must be made by the surgeon in charge

II. Notification of Death
   A. Surgeon responsibilities
      1. Notification of family/next of kin
   B. Circulating nurse's responsibilities
      1. Notification of the cardiac manager or acting nursing supervisor
      2. Notification of the death of the patient to the intensive care unit
      3. Notification of clergy, if requested
      4. Coordinating the postmortem care
      5. Notification of the coroner

III. Postmortem Care
   A. Care of the body
      1. Removal of all tubes and catheters once the coroner has given permission
      2. Cleaning the body
      3. Replacement of dentures
      4. Labeling of the body for proper identification
   B. Family considerations
      1. The family may request viewing of the body.
         a. The body is transported to a clean, private area of the surgical department for viewing.
         b. The healthcare team provides support to the family, as needed.
   C. The body is prepared for transport to the morgue.
      1. The body is placed in a body bag.
      2. The body is transported to the morgue in a special morgue transport vehicle.

IV. Documentation
   A. Surgeon's responsibilities
      1. Completed patient record
      2. Completed death certificate
      3. Assistance with obtaining the appropriate consents from the family
   B. Circulating nurse's responsibilities
      1. Completed surgical record
      2. Completed nursing notes
         a. Sequence of events
         b. Time of death

           c. Name of surgeon who pronounced the patient
           d. Name of the medical examiner giving permission to proceed with the postmortem care
           e. Completed variance report sheet
           f. CPR record, if indicated

V. Special Considerations of Intraoperative Mortality
    A. The team is aware of special consents requesting "No CPR" orders, preoperatively.
    B. Permission must be received from the medical examiner before postmortem care can be performed.
    C. The body remains on the surgical table with all tubes and lines in place until the approval for removal has been received.
    D. Postmortem care is not given if it conflicts with the religious beliefs of the patient.

VI. Grieving Process
    A. Family
        1. The team is supportive and respective of all family wishes.
        2. The family is assisted with the disposition of the body and personal belongings.
    B. Staff
        1. The staff members are given time to express their feelings of death.
           a. Acknowledgment of efforts is reinforced.
           b. Limitations are shared.

VII. Clinical Indicators for Evaluation
    A. Number of intraoperative mortalities
    B. Staffing education pertaining to the postmortem process
        1. Postmortem care is carried out efficiently and effectively according to specific guidelines.
           a. The body is properly prepared and identified.
           b. All appropriate documentation is completed.
           c. The family is supported.
        2. Staff feelings toward death and dying
           a. Effective coping mechanisms

Surgical Intervention of the Neonate

Neonates are unique with specific individual needs. Advanced knowledge of these needs is imperative for the provision of optimal surgical intervention. Using the nursing process of assessing, planning, implementing, and evaluating to meet the individual needs of each neonate is critical throughout the perioperative period.

The perioperative care of the neonate revolves around the infant's weight and age, type of defect, and conservation of body heat. The weight of these infants can range from 450 grams (1 pound) to 10 to 12 pounds.

The surgical procedure may be carried out in the operating room or the neonatal intensive care unit dependent on the infant's condition.

An isolette is used to transport neonates to surgery. The isolette has an oxygen tank and an air bag attached. The gases are blended to prevent retrolental fibroplasia or retinopathy of prematurity. Retinopathy of prematurity is the vasoconstriction of the retinal capillaries that can lead to retinal detachment and scarring associated with the use of 100% oxygen. It can result in irreversible blindness.

A blender for both tanks, transport ventilator, and an EKG monitor should also accompany the isolette. Extra supplies such as blood pressure cuffs, oxygen masks, IV tubing, and ambu bags are kept at the bottom of the cart for emergencies. These supplies must be available in a variety of sizes to accommodate the specific needs of the individual neonate, depending on his or her weight, size, and age.

The infant's transport should be achieved as quickly as possible to prevent the infant from receiving the dry air in the isolette any longer than necessary. When an infant is intubated, a very small endotracheal tube is used. It is easy for secretions to plug the tubes when exposed to dry air. Transport humidifiers are not used on isolettes because the water chamber may tip during transport, sending the water through the tubing to the patient. After transport, the isolette is moved outside the surgical suite and connected to an electrical outlet to maintain the heat and be ready for transport when surgery is completed.

These infants have a much larger body weight surface area relative to their body weight and have great difficulty in producing and conserving heat. Heat is lost through radiation, convection, evaporation, and conduction.

The temperature of the surgery suite is set higher to prevent heat loss through radiation and convection. Warming lights, kept at a distance of 27 inches from the baby to prevent burns, are used to conserve heat. A warming blanket is placed under the sheet of the OR table to prevent heat loss from conduction.

Immediate perioperative assessment of the neonate includes

A. The infant's weight and age
B. NPO status, usually consisting of 6 hours of clear liquid followed by 4 hours of NPO

C. Presence, location, and patency of peripheral IVS
D. Presence of hemodynamic monitoring lines, that is CVP, arterial lines
E. Lab values: The neonate's hemoglobin, hematocrit, and white blood counts are higher than in adults. The normal range for hemoglobin is 14–18 grams. Hematocrit ranges from 45% to 50%. White blood cells are usually 20,000.
F. Assessment pertaining to respiratory, circulatory, integumentary, nutritional, and levels of mentation
G. Consents for surgical intervention

It is critical to ensure that vitamin K was given after delivery to prevent hemorrhage during the surgical procedure. One milligram of vitamin K is given intramuscularly at birth for clotting. Vitamin K catalyzes the synthesis of prothrombin in the liver. In adults, vitamin K is synthesized by the intestinal flora, but a newborn's intestinal tract is sterile. Vitamin K is not present for prothrombin formation until the newborn's intestinal flora is established, usually in about 4 days.

Fluid replacement is monitored closely to prevent fluid overload. The I.V. preparation for the neonates is usually 250- or 500-ml bags of dextrose and lactated Ringer's solution. Glucose stores are rapidly depleted from neonates and must be replaced. Intravenous line drip chambers, called buretrols, are always used and filled with only 30 ml of fluid. Special microbore tubing, which holds about 1.5 ml of fluid, is also used. It is extremely important to ensure that there are no air bubbles in the I.V. tubing. Even the smallest air bubble could cause an air embolism. Tiny arm boards are used to prevent the I.V. line from kinking and inadvertent dislodgement as the baby moves. Small infusion or syringe pumps are used to monitor fluid replacement.

Extreme care is taken during the transfer from the isolette to the OR table to prevent the dislodgement of the I.V. lines. Noninvasive monitoring equipment is applied. Pediatric EKG pads and a blood pressure cuff are positioned. Paper tape instead of plastic tape is used for reinforcement. Paper tape causes less trauma to the infant's fragile skin.

The normal heart rate of these infants ranges from 110 to 160 beats per minute. The blood pressure is not usually higher than 80 mm Hg.

A Doppler ultrasound may be placed over the radial artery to be used as backup in case the arterial line fails during the procedure. A pulse oximeter is used on all neonates to measure the arterial oxygen saturation and give continuous pulse readout. The pulse oximeter is taped on the infant's hand or foot because the fingers or toes are usually too small for the probe.

A rectal probe is inserted for continual temperature monitoring. A bladder drainage tube is used only if the infant's condition and procedure warrant. Approximate urine measurements are accomplished by use of a pedi-bag that collects urine. If urine measurement is critical, a small feeding tube is used to drain the bladder. When all monitors are in place, the circulating nurse places a pediatric electrosurgical dispersement pad on the infant's back. This is usually the largest area of the neonate's body to ground. The infant's legs and arms are wrapped with cotton padding to prevent excessive heat loss. The nerves and pressure areas are padded using foam pads or small nonradiopaque sponges. The head is large in proportion to the rest of the neonate's tiny body. Foam padding is placed beneath the head to prevent pressure damage. The head may be covered with a small stockinette for warmth. The extremities are protected with emesis basins cut in half and placed over the hands and feet.

To prevent excessive heat loss from evaporation and conduction, the prep solutions are warmed approximately 5 minutes before the surgical prep is performed. To decrease heat loss by evaporation, it is best to prep dry by squeezing out the prep sponges. After the prep is completed, the posterior side of the infant is assessed to ensure that prep solutions have not pooled, predisposing the infant to chemical burns.

The neonates are draped immediately after the prep is completed to conserve body heat.

The surgical team is careful not to lean or bear weight on the infant's tiny structure.

Small incisions and small anatomical structures require small, delicate instruments. Instruments must be passed gently so that the surgeon does not have to take his eyes off of the sterile field. Retraction must be done very carefully to prevent lacerations that could occur by pulling too hard on the infant's organs.

Warm irrigating solutions are used on neonates. The amount and temperature of the irrigation are extremely important. Hot irrigating fluids can burn the infant's fragile tissue. Warm sponges, wrung dry, are used to prevent conduction and evaporative heat loss. Careful and accurate calculations are used to determine blood loss and fluid replacement. Sponges are weighed after they are discarded from the field. Suction from the operative field is collected in a special reservoir that accurately measures tiny amounts of fluid. The normal blood volume in a neonate is 80–85 ml kg.

The surgeons wear headlights and surgical loops for better visualization.

Surgical incisions in the neonates are closed with an undyed, absorbable suture rather than skin staples.

Frequent communication with the family regarding the neonate's progress is important.

After the drapes are removed, the circulator is responsible for assisting with the dressings, removing the dispersive electrode pad gently, checking for possible burns, and assisting the anesthesiologist with the transfer. The infant is transferred from the OR table to the warmed isolette and returned to the neonatal unit.

Risk Management

chapter 10

■ Cardiac Surgery: Policy: Safety Reports

Cardiac surgery's policy is that a monthly safety report be submitted to the hospital's safety program for the purposes of

1. Reporting, investigating, and evaluating incidents
2. Hazard prevention and surveillance
   a. To prevent personal injury
   b. To prevent damage to equipment
   c. To prevent damage to facilities

Cardiac Surgery: Nursing Procedure: Safety Reports

Quality Outcome: Monthly safety reports are completed for review and evaluation by the hospital safety committee.

Performed by: Cardiac team member and cardiac surgery manager

General Statement: All cardiac surgical team members adhere to the hospital's safety program. A cardiac team member participates in the hospital's safety committee to keep the team updated on periodic reviews of fire and disaster drills and safety educational programs.

Equipment: Safety report sheets

Steps:	Rationale:

1. The cardiac manager prepares a safety report monthly, including but not limited to the following information:
  a. Documentation of safety inservices
  b. Report of safety hazards
  c. Follow-up on safety hazards
  d. Occurrences pertaining to the patient, staff, or institution
	The hospital safety committee reviews, evaluates, and makes recommendations for safety procedures and occurrences.

2. A cardiac surgery team member is a representative on the hospital's safety committee.	The cardiac surgical team member is a liaison for the cardiac surgical team and relays critical information regarding safety drills and plans for fire, earthquake, and other disasters.
3. A monthly safety inservice is given. The agenda, attendance, and date are documented.	Each member is trained and prepared to carry out special duties in case of emergencies and disasters and in recognizing the hazards of the work environment.

Cardiac Surgery: Policy: Housekeeping of the Cardiac Surgical Suite

Cardiac surgery's policy is that a specific plan is established and carried out between the housekeeping department and the surgery housekeeping staff to maintain an environment conducive to safe surgical intervention with preventative measures to eliminate microorganisms from the operating room suite.

Cardiac Surgery: Nursing Procedure: Environmental Control of the Cardiac Surgical Suite

Quality Outcome: The environment of the cardiac surgical suite is controlled and monitored to facilitate safe surgical intervention by establishing preventative measures to eliminate microorganisms.

Performed by: Hospital housekeeping staff, surgery housekeeping staff, and cardiac team members

General Statement: Sanitation practices should provide a safe, clean environment for the surgical patient and personnel. All surgical cases are considered potentially contaminated.

Equipment: A hospital-approved cleaning disinfectant; housekeeping equipment; OSHA-approved sharp, laundry, and disposable waste receptacles

Steps:	Rationale:
1. Before the first procedure of the day, furniture, surgical lights, and equipment are damp dusted.	Between 90% and 99% of viable microbial contaminants from the air and other sources are deposited on the horizontal surfaces in the operating room.
2. Damp dusting is accomplished using clean, lint-free material moistened with a hospital-grade disinfectant.	Proper cleaning of these flat surfaces helps to control airborne microorganisms.
3. The temperature and humidity of the surgical suite are monitored. The temperature should be maintained between 20 and 24 degrees centigrade and the humidity at a maximum of 50%.	The temperature and humidity are regulated to reduce metabolic demands on the patient, reduce bacterial growth, suppress static electricity, and provide surgeon comfort while operating.
4. During the surgical procedure, efforts are directed at confining contamination with prompt cleanup of organic debris and blood using an approved hospital disinfectant.	Contaminated surfaces shall be cleaned immediately or as soon as feasible, maintaining a safe, clean environment.

Steps:	Rationale:
5. Contaminated, disposable items are discarded into a covered, impervious container, color coded and labeled. Laundry is handled as little as possible and bagged in containers that are impervious, color coded, and labeled. Suction liners are closed and disposed of according to hospital policy.	Follows OSHA regulations to prevent cross-contamination and safe handling of contaminated materials.
6. All blood bags, body fluids, and tissue specimens are placed in a clean, impervious container and sealable bag for transport to the lab.	Inanimate objects soiled with blood or body fluids may potentially infect healthcare workers. Sealable bags are used to prevent leakage of fluids during handling, storage, and transport.
7. All personnel working or observing in the cardiac surgical suite wear personal protective equipment from the beginning of the surgical procedure, continuing through the decontamination of the surgical suite.	Protective attire is worn to protect the staff members' skin, clothing, and mucous membranes against contact with blood or other potentially infectious body fluids.
8. The scrub nurse places all of the dirty instruments in basins containing a hospital-approved disinfectant and covered for transport to the instrument-reprocessing area. Sharp containers are covered and removed after each case. Terminal cleaning of furniture, floors, and equipment is accomplished.	Contaminated items are covered to prevent inadvertent exposure of personnel to infectious material. All contaminated work surfaces are decontaminated after completion of the procedure.
9. Terminal cleaning is done at the end of the day per the hospital housekeeping schedule and documented for references and evaluation.	Recordkeeping of the sanitation process is required for OSHA.

Steps:	Rationale:
10. The cardiac manager and the housekeeping manager meet every month to evaluate the sanitation process for the cardiac surgical suite.	The work site is maintained in a clean and sanitary condition.
11. A monthly cleaning schedule is designed for the cardiac surgical suite with the housekeeping department.	Sanitation is essential to reduce the possibility of contamination of the patient, personnel, and operating room.

Standard of Care: Environmental Control of the Cardiac Surgical Suite

I. Housekeeping Schedule
   A. Written outline of specific duties
      1. Operating room cleaning staff
      2. Housekeeping staff
   B. Terminal cleaning schedule
      1. Before the start of first case
      2. Between cases
      3. End of day
      4. Weekly
      5. Monthly
   C. Documentation of terminal cleaning and evaluation
II. Climate Control
   A. Air conduit system
      1. Filters cleaned and changed routinely
      2. Room temperature kept between 60 and 70 degrees
      3. Humidity between 35% and 50%
   B. Waste removal protocol
      1. Soiled laundry
      2. Solid waste
         a. Clean trash
         b. Contaminated trash
      3. Dirty instrument processing
   C. Physical considerations
      1. Traffic to a minimum
      2. Doors to the surgical suite kept closed
      3. Limit observers
   D. Clinical indicators for evaluation
      1. General cleanliness of room
         a. Monthly evaluations with the housekeeping department
      2. Staff education
         a. Staff compliance
      3. Patient outcomes
         a. Infection rate of postoperative cardiac patients

Cardiac Surgery: Policy: Electrical Safety

Cardiac surgery's policy is that

1. Electromedical equipment used in the cardiac surgical suite is to be included in an appropriate inspection and maintenance program to assure the safe operation of the equipment. Records of routine maintenance or repair of equipment will be kept by the cardiac surgical manager and the biomedical electronic department.
2. All personnel using the electrical devices will be instructed in their proper use and care. Instruction manuals available.
3. All staff is able to locate and identify the electrical line isolation monitor and alarms.
4. A procedure is available for deactivating an electrical alarm warning.
5. All staff is aware of how to access the emergency power system.
6. All personnel must be introduced to possible hazards of burn, shock, explosion, fire, injury, and death. All personnel are instructed in BCLS.
7. Equipment is examined before use.
8. Electromedical equipment with patient leads or other connectors intended to be attached directly to the heart or to an invasive conductive pathway shall be provided with special electrically isolated leads.
9. Any extension cords used must be grounded.
10. Room humidity is maintained at between 35% and 50%.

Cardiac Surgery: Nursing Procedure: Electrical Hazard Prevention

Quality Outcome: To assure the safe operation of electrical equipment that is in direct contact with the patient in cardiac surgery

Performed by: Perfusionist, hemodynamic monitoring specialist, circulating nurse, scrub nurse, and biomedical engineers

General Statement: Electrical equipment shall be inspected and tested daily before use. Safe practices are established to decrease potential hazards associated with the use of electrical equipment.

Equipment: All standard electrical equipment used in the cardiac surgical suite.

Steps:	Rationale:
1. The cord length on all electrical equipment should be inspected for frays or damage.	Damaged cords present a shock hazard to the patient and personnel.
2. The cord length is appropriate for the intended use.	A longer cord prevents the hazard of tripping over the cords.
3. The electrical outlets are checked for damage and reported immediately to the bioengineering department. The equipment is exchanged if damage is present.	Damaged outlets may contribute to excessive leakage of electrical current.
4. The isolated power system is checked. If the line isolation monitor alarms, indicating a potential hazard, the last piece of electrical equipment plugged into an electrical source is unplugged. If the alarm continues, each piece of electrical equipment is unplugged, one at a time, until the alarm stops. The biomedical engineer is called to check for the electrical current leakage.	The warning system indicates when inadvertent grounding of isolated circuits has occurred and alerts personnel to a dangerous situation. The faulty equipment can be identified.

Steps:	Rationale:
5. Personnel are educated in specific equipment utilization, maintenance, and safety. Recommended practices published by the manufacturer are followed.	The manufacturer provides safety guidelines and utilization instructions for the use of its equipment.
6. All electrical equipment is included in an appropriate preventive maintenance program.	Equipment is maintained according to the manufacturers' guidelines with routine electrical inspection completed at regular intervals according to hospital policy.
7. All new electrical equipment is inspected by the biomedical department before use.	Safety requirements are met.
8. Liquids are not set on electrical equipment.	Liquids could cause an internal short circuit if spilled.

Cardiac Surgery: Standard of Care: Electrical Safety

I. Inspection of Equipment
   A. Biomedical department inspection before the first use
   B. Daily inspection before use
      1. Cord length
      2. Cord integrity
      3. Electrical outlets
      4. Functioning capability of the equipment
   C. Quarterly maintenance inspection by the biomedical department
II. Staff Education
   A. Staff is educated on the function and use of all electrical equipment
      1. The recommended practices from the manufacturer are used as guidelines.
      2. All equipment is properly grounded.
         a. Dispersive electrode pads are safely positioned.
      3. Plugs are removed from their electrical source at the plug level, not pulled by the cord.
      4. Equipment is turned off when staff is plugging or unplugging the unit(s).
      5. The staff is able to locate and identify the electrical isolation alarm and know the steps to isolate the area of electrical current leakage.
      6. Electrocautery pencils are kept in their protective holder on the surgical field.
   B. Staff awareness of potential hazards
      1. Cord length
      2. Cord integrity
      3. Electrical outlet integrity
      4. Ignition sources
      5. Liquids placed on an electrical unit
      6. Electrical burns
      7. Cardiac arrest
III. Line Isolation Monitor Alarms
   A. Alarm is set off when there is electrical current leakage or failure.
      1. The last piece of equipment plugged into an electrical source is unplugged.
      2. Electrical equipment is unplugged one at a time in order to see where the leakage is occurring.
      3. Biomedical engineering is called.
IV. Emergency Electrical Power Supply
   A. Backup emergency battery supply

        B. Emergency overhead surgical lights
        C. Flashlights
        D. Hand crank on the heart–lung machine
V.   Safety Reports
        A. Completed monthly
            1. A representative of the cardiac team serves on the hospital safety committee
                a. Unsafe occurrences reported
                b. Evaluation and follow-up
                c. Documentation of safety meetings
VI. Clinical Indicators for Evaluation
        A. Patient safety
        B. Staff safety
        C. Electrical occurrences
        D. Electrical maintenance
        E. Staff education and training pertaining to electrical safety
        F. Monthly documentation for the safety committee
        G. Periodic safety checks for the availability of the emergency battery backup system

Cardiac Surgery: Policy: Electrocautery Utilization

Cardiac surgery's policy is that the following criteria be met when using electrocautery unit(s) during a cardiac surgical procedure:

1. The patients are properly grounded using the hospital-approved grounding pad, one per electrocautery unit used.
2. Proper placement of the grounding pad is accomplished to prevent interference with the surgical field, cardiac arrest due to electrical interference with the cardiac monitoring electrodes, or patient burns. The grounding site placement is documented on the operative record.
3. Cardiac monitoring electrodes are placed as far away from the operative field as possible. The sites of the monitoring electrodes are assessed preoperatively and postoperatively.
4. The condition of the grounding pad placement site, both preoperatively and postoperatively, is documented on the surgical record.
5. The serial number(s) of the electrocautery unit(s) and the power settings used is documented on the surgical record.
6. A protective, nonconductive holster is used for the cautery pencil on the surgical field when not in use.
7. Two electrocautery units are used when performing a dual procedure to prevent activation of both cautery pencils simultaneously, increasing the risk of patient burns.

Cardiac Surgery: Nursing Procedure: Electrocautery Safety

Quality Outcome: Electrocautery safety is assured perioperatively through staff education on electrical safety and prevention, maintenance, and inspection of electrocautery equipment, appropriate patient grounding, and appropriate use and care of the electrosurgical pencil(s) on the surgical field.

Performed by: Licensed and cardiac surgical staff

General Statement: The incidence of electrical burns or the potential for a cardiac arrest due to electrical interference of an electrically monitored patient is diminished with proper EKG electrode placement and electrosurgical dispersement grounding pad placement. One electrosurgical dispersement pad is needed for each electrocautery unit used. CABG surgical procedures require two electrocautery units, necessitating the need for two electrosurgical dispersement pads.

Electrosurgical pencils used on the sterile field are contained in a nonconductive holster when not in use. The tip is kept free of debris during surgery. Postoperatively, the tip is removed and disposed of properly.

Equipment: Electrocautery unit(s), electrosurgical dispersement pads with cable, and electrosurgical pencil and holster

Steps:	Rationale:
1. All staff members are educated in the appropriate electrical safety and proper use of the electrocautery unit used in cardiac surgery.	Instruction and return demonstration in proper usage assist in preventing injury and extend the life of the equipment.
Equipment manuals are available for reference.	Equipment manuals provide operational, safety, and maintenance guidelines.
2. Preoperatively, the circulating nurse inspects the electrocautery unit(s) to be used. The unit(s) is plugged into the electrical outlet.	The equipment is available and functioning before the start of the surgical procedure. Broken wire or frays can deviate current flows. Incomplete circuitry may lead to patient injury.

Steps:	Rationale:
3. The patient is positioned on the surgical table, and cardiac monitoring electrodes are applied laterally to the arms and hips bilaterally and the left lateral chest wall, as far away from the operative field as possible.	The position of the electrodes is dependent on optimal surgical exposure permitting well-defined cardiac monitoring and prevention of electrical dispersement from the electrocautery pencil.

4. After induction, the circulating nurse assesses the site(s) for the electrosurgical dispersement pad(s). The grounding sites must meet the following requirements:
  a. The dispersive electrode pad is placed as close to the operative site as possible.
  b. The grounding site is free of hair and scar tissue.
  c. Bony prominences and areas over any metal implants are avoided.
  d. The dispersive electrode pad must be placed on a clean, dry surface, maintaining uniform body contact.
	Placing the dispersive electrode close to the surgical site minimizes the current through the body.
	
	Hair and scar tissue tend to adhere poorly and act as insulation. Pressure points cause current concentration.
	
	The metal implants could divert current.
	
	The amount of surface area affects heat buildup at the dispersive site.

5. The dispersive electrode pad for the median sternotomy is placed on the patient's posterior flank, or on the upper arm, if available.	The dispersive electrode pad is placed as close to the surgical site as possible without interfering with the surgical site.
6. The dispersive electrode pad for use in the vein-harvesting procedure, if applicable, is placed on the buttock.	Same as above.
7. Care is taken not to place the dispersive electrode pads side by side.	Dispersive electrode pads that are placed in close proximity to each other may cause arching of electrical current with subsequent incidence of patient burns.

Cardiac Surgery: Nursing Procedure: Electrocautery Safety

Steps:	Rationale:
8. The cable(s) from the dispersive electrode pad(s) is connected to its prospective electrocautery units. The electrocautery pencil from the field is connected to the proper terminal on the electrocautery unit. The cautery pencil is not attached to the unit until the dispersement electrode pad has been connected to the unit.	Incomplete circuitry and unintentional activation may result in patient injury.
9. The electrocautery unit is turned on. The power setting is calibrated according to the physician's preference. The power setting is documented on the surgical record.	The surgeon is aware of the cautery settings to prevent unnecessary damage to tissue. Perioperative care is documented.
10. During the surgical procedure, the scrub nurse keeps the tip of the cautery pencil free of debris. The cautery pencil is placed in a clean, dry holster when not in use. Postoperatively, the tip from the electrocautery pencil is removed and disposed of properly.	The cautery tip is cleaned to facilitate the conduction of heat. It prevents the possibility of patient burns. The cautery tip is treated as a sharp item and is disposed of safely.
11. Postoperatively, the circulating nurse removes the dispersive electrode. Assessment of the skin at the dispersive electrode site and under the cardiac monitoring electrodes is performed. The circulating nurse documents the following on the surgical record: a. Skin integrity before and after electrocautery use b. Serial numbers of the electrocautery units c. Power settings used during electrocautery use	Assessment will allow evaluation of the skin for possible injury. Surgical documentation is completed for care rendered. Identification numbers permit documentation for inspections and tracking of equipment problems.

Steps:	Rationale:
12. If an adverse skin reaction occurs, the circulating nurse informs the physician, initiates an incident report, and sends the electrosurgical unit, cautery pencil, and dispersive electrode pad to the biomedical service.	Retaining the electrical equipment in question allows for a complete systems check to determine system integrity.
13. The power on the electrosurgical unit(s) is turned off and cleaned with a damp cloth.	The electrocautery unit(s) must be kept clean and dry.

Cardiac Surgery: Policy: Protective Attire

Cardiac surgery's policy is that all personnel working or observing in the cardiac surgical suite wear impervious gowns and face masks, gloves, shoe covers, and protective eye shields at all times during a surgical procedure, reducing the risk of exposure to blood or body fluids that may contain potentially infectious microorganisms.

Cardiac Surgery: Nursing Procedure: Protective Attire

Quality Outcome: Protective attire worn by the cardiac staff decreases the risk of exposure to blood or body fluids that may contain infectious micro-organisms.

Performed by: All team members participating in a cardiac surgical case and any individual observing the procedure

General Statement: Guidelines are established and enforced regarding protective attire worn by the team during a cardiac surgical procedure. The protective equipment is effective in preventing the penetration of blood and other potentially infectious materials. The equipment is accessible and conveniently located inside the cardiac surgical suite.

Equipment: Impervious gowns, rubber gloves, face shields/goggles, fluid-resistant surgical masks, and shoe covers

Steps:	Rationale:
1. The scrub nurse places protective eyewear over her eyes before the surgical hand scrub. The eyewear must completely cover all sides of the eyes. The surgical mask is in place.	Eyes are protected whenever splashes, splatter, or sprays are reasonably expected and eye, nose, or mouth contamination can be reasonably anticipated.
2. The scrub nurse dons the sterile, impervious gown and gloves to prepare the instrumentation needed for the procedure.	The appropriate attire is worn for the surgical procedure.
3. The circulating nurse, hemodynamic monitoring specialist, and perfusionist don impervious gowns and gloves as soon as the patient enters the surgical suite. Eye shields/goggles are placed over the eyes.	Proper attire prevents exposure to blood and body fluids.

Steps:	Rationale:
4. The soiled gown and gloves are removed and exchanged for new sets, as needed, throughout the surgical procedure and are properly disposed. The gown is removed first, with the gloves to follow, pulling the gloves inside out. Hands are washed after removing gloves.	Prevents contamination of blood and body fluids to other staff members. Gloves are replaced as soon as practical when contaminated or as soon as is feasible if they are torn or punctured or when their ability to function as a barrier is compromised.
5. Staff must remove their protective attire before leaving the surgical suite in a designated area or container.	OSHA requirements.
6. The protective attire can be discarded after the instruments have been removed to the decontamination area and the room has been cleaned according to hospital policy.	Exposure prevention. All equipment and environmental and working surfaces shall be cleaned and decontaminated after contact with blood or other potentially infectious materials.

Standard of Care: Cardiac Surgery: Risk Management

I. Work Practice Controls
   A. Exposure control
      1. Plan created to protect employees/nonemployees from blood-borne pathogens
         a. Determination of what tasks put employees at risk
         b. Schedule of implementation for the methods of compliance
         c. Hepatitis B vaccination
            1. Employees may refuse the vaccination but must sign the OSHA-required waiver indicating their refusal
         d. Training and inservicing
            1. Current policies and procedures are accessible to all staff members.
            2. Training must be provided to staff at the time of the initial assignment and repeated every 12 months or when changes of tasks or procedures occur.
         e. Exposure procedure
            1. All exposure incidents must be reported, investigated, and documented.
            2. Medical evaluation is completed.
            3. Follow-up plan and evaluation
         f. Record keeping
            1. Incidents
            2. Staff training
   B. Engineering control
      1. Devices used to minimize employee exposure by removing or isolating blood-borne pathogen hazards from the workplace
         a. Protective attire is worn by the staff and observers during the surgical procedure. This attire is accessible and conveniently located. The attire is effective in preventing the penetration of blood and other potentially infectious materials.
            1. Impervious gowns
            2. Fluid-resistant masks
            3. Protective eye shields/goggles
            4. Shoe covers
            5. Disposable gloves
         b. Handling of sharps
            1. Needles are not recapped, bent, removed, broken, or sheared.

    2. Sharps are disposed of in an approved sharps container and properly disposed of after each case.
    3. A "hands-free" sharp zone is used if possible during the surgical procedure.
   c. Specimen handling
    1. Specimens are placed in an approved sealed container that prevents leaks or spills of its contents.
    2. Specimen containers are placed in sealed bags for transport to the lab.
   d. Housekeeping
    1. Frequent hand washing
     a. After removal of gloves
    2. All contaminated work surfaces will be decontaminated after completion of procedures and immediately, or as soon as feasible, after any spill of blood or other potentially infectious material.
    3. Equipment used must be decontaminated before next use, shipping, or servicing.
    4. Contaminated laundry
     a. Bagged or contained in the location where it was used
     b. Handled as little as possible
     c. Labeled with the hazard sign
II. Clinical Indicators for Evaluation
 A. Exposure control plan meets OSHA regulations
 B. Staff education
  1. Staff compliance with the regulations.
 C. Incidence of exposure
 D. Follow-up and evaluation of incidence

Cardiac Surgery: Policy: Surgical Consents

Cardiac surgery's policy is that the following informed consents be obtained pre-operatively, according to the state, federal, and hospital regulations, including but not limited to

1. Consent for the surgical procedure
2. Request and consent for the administration of anesthesia
3. Disclosure and consent for transfusion of blood/blood products
4. Refusal of consents are obtained, if applicable

Cardiac Surgery: Nursing Procedure: Surgical Consents

Quality Outcome: Valid consents are obtained and assessed for all cardiac surgical patients receiving treatment, diagnostic, and surgical procedures.

Performed by: Cardiac surgeon, cardiac surgery office, and circulating nurse

General Statement: The circulating nurse reviews the chart before the transfer of the cardiac surgical patient to the surgical suite. The consents are documented according to policy and appropriate for the surgical procedure to be performed.

Equipment: Appropriate consent forms

Steps:	Rationale:

1. The circulating nurse reviews the chart for the appropriate consents before the transfer of the patient to the surgical suite, including but not limited to
   a. Consent for the surgical procedure
   b. Consent for anesthesia and invasive line placement
   c. Disclosure and consent for transfusion of blood and blood products
   d. Refusal of treatment consents, if applicable
   e. Special procedure consents, if applicable
	The circulating nurse ensures that the informed consents are obtained before the surgical procedure. The patient maintains the right of self-determination of his or her own person.

2. The consents are assessed for complete documentation, including but not limited to
   a. Consent for the correct surgical procedure
   b. Signature of the patient
   c. Date of signature
	The consents are documented according to hospital policy to minimize liability for the patient, staff, and institution.

Steps:	Rationale:
3. The circulating nurse notifies the surgeon of any discrepancies. If a consent has been omitted, another consent can be obtained if the patient has not had any narcotics within the last 4 hours.	A consent is not valid if signed after a patient has had any narcotics within the last 4 hours.
4. The circulating nurse informs the team of any refusal of treatment consents.	Notification of the team of refusal of treatment consents facilitates the intraoperative plan of care.
5. If a patient requires emergency surgery and is unable to sign his or her own consent, the circulating nurse ensures that the consent is signed by the cardiac surgeons.	Two physicians' signatures are required in an extreme emergency for the consent to be valid.

Cardiac Surgery: Nursing Procedure: Surgical Consents

Standard of Care: Cardiac Surgery: Surgical Consents

I. Consent Goals
   A. Maintain the patient's right of self-determination over his or her own person
      1. The patient has the right to refuse treatment.
         a. The patient must have an adequate understanding of his or her condition.
         b. The patient must understand the consequence of denying treatment.
         c. The patient must sign a refusal of treatment consent form.
   B. Ensure that an informed consent is obtained before the surgical procedure
      1. Documented according to policy
      2. Appropriate for the surgical procedure to be performed
      3. Minimize liability
         a. Patient
         b. Staff
         c. Institution
II. Pertinent Consents
   A. Consent for a surgical procedure
   B. Request and consent for administration of anesthesia
   C. Disclosure and consent for transfusion of blood/blood products
   D. Refusal of treatment consent, if applicable
   E. Special procedure consents completed at the same time as the original surgical procedure, if applicable
      1. Placement of a permanent pacemaker
      2. Placement of an intra-aortic balloon
      3. Placement of a VAD
      4. Placement of an internal cardioverter defibrillator
      5. Transesophageal echocardiography
III. Responsibility of the Surgeon
   A. Inform the patient
   B. Obtain the consent
   C. Emergently
      1. The signatures of two physicians are acceptable.
IV. Responsibility of the Circulating Nurse
   A. Ensure that the appropriate consents have been obtained.
   B. Ensure that the consents are documented according to hospital, state, and federal regulations.

C. Assess the patient's level of understanding.
       D. Ensure that the surgical team is aware of any discrepancies.
              1. Refusal of treatment with blood/blood products is made known to the team.
V.   Special Consents
       A. Consents for photographs
       B. Consents for observers in the surgical suite
VI.   Clinical Indicators for Evaluation
       A. Staff education concerning consents
              1. Written policies and procedures concerning informed consents
                     a. Scheduled and emergent
       B. Monitoring the standard of care
              1. Chart review preoperatively
                     a. Appropriate consent for the surgical procedure
                     b. Eligibility of the patient to sign a consent
              2. Scheduled procedure
              3. Emergent procedure
              4. Variance reporting
                     a. Omissions
                     b. Improper documentation
                     c. Patient's level of understanding

Cardiac Surgery: Policy: Perioperative Documentation of Cardiac Surgical Procedures

Cardiac surgery's policy is that the following documentation be completed and tracked to facilitate case management of cardiac surgical procedures with the capability to evaluate the care rendered, including but not limited to:

1. Perioperative documentation
2. Statistical documentation
3. Implantation documentation, if applicable
4. Continuing education of the staff
5. Electrical safety
6. Inventory of supplies, instrumentation, and equipment
7. Policies and procedures relating to cardiac surgery
8. Surgical suite housekeeping
9. Infection control
10. Variance reports
11. CPR record, if applicable
12. Intensive care documentation sheet

Cardiac Surgery: Nursing Procedure: Perioperative Documentation of Cardiac Surgical Procedures

Quality Outcome: Complete documentation of the perioperative period is documented with statistical records maintained to evaluate the care rendered.

Performed by: Cardiac surgeon, cardiac anesthesiologist, perfusionist, circulating nurse, and cardiac manager

General Statement: Each member of the team is responsible for specific documentation of the care rendered to each patient perioperatively. Guidelines are established to facilitate the documentation process and to ensure that documentation is complete.

Equipment: Corresponding documentation records

Steps:	Rationale:
1. The circulating nurse documents that the preoperative checklist is completed, noting any discrepancies or abnormalities before transferring the patient to the surgical suite.	Ensures that the surgical procedure is not delayed and facilitates the intraoperative plan of care.
2. The circulating nurse completes the surgical record and fluid flow sheet. The patient's name, surgeon's name, procedure performed, team members involved, and any complications are logged in the procedure log book.	Intraoperative documentation of the surgical procedure and patient's response to the procedure is documented. The procedure log is useful in tracking trends over time.
3. The cardiac anesthesiologist completes the anesthesia record.	The patient's response to anesthesia and the agents used are documented for further reference.
4. The perfusionist completes the perfusion record and the mortality risk documentation sheet.	Documentation of cardiopulmonary bypass is completed. The record is used for further reference, if needed. The mortality risk sheet assists with the tracking of the acuity of the patient population.

Steps:	Rationale:
5. Documentation is completed for any variance, that is, cardiac arrest, delay in the surgical procedure, or unavailability of supplies.	Facilitates the evaluation of care rendered.

6. All implants are logged on the surgical record and implantation log book. Information includes but is not limited to
  a. Name of manufacturer
  b. Type of implant
  c. Size and model and serial numbers
  d. Location of implant
  e. Date received
  f. Date implanted
  g. Expiration date, if applicable
	Assists with inventory management and tracking of implants for future reference, if a problem arises.

7. The intensive care documentation sheet is completed before the patient leaves the surgical suite.	Facilitates the transition of the patient from surgery to the intensive care unit. Continuity of care is accomplished.
8. The cardiac manager manages documentation pertaining to the staff's continuing education, inventory of supplies and equipment, housekeeping, safety, and infection control.	Specific record keeping is essential to meet JCAHO's requirements and to be able to track and use statistical data to evaluate and maintain optimal levels of quality control.
9. Policies and procedures are written, evaluated, and revised annually. The policies and procedures are easily accessible for all staff members.	Meets JCAHO, state, and federal requirements.

Standard of Care: Cardiac Surgery: Perioperative Documentation of Cardiac Surgical Procedures

I. Perioperative Documentation
   A. Preoperative surgical checklist
   B. Surgical record
   C. Perfusion record
   D. Anesthesia record
   E. Fluid flow record
   F. Mortality risk record
   G. Cardiac surgical case log
   H. Intensive care documentation sheet
II. Records Tracking Statistical Data
   A. Number, types, and duration of surgical procedures
   B. Environmental data
   C. Utilization of staffing, surgical suite, supplies, and equipment
   D. Infection control
   E. Implant log
   F. Safety
   G. Inventory of equipment, supplies, and instrumentation
III. Staff Education
   A. Minutes and agendas of meetings
   B. Skills checklist
   C. Knowledge of policies and procedures
IV. Clinical Indicators for Evaluation
   A. Complete documentation
   B. JCAHO, federal, and state compliant
   C. Evaluation of trends

Cardiac Surgery: Policy: Patient Transfer Report

Cardiac surgery's policy is that complete documentation of the surgical procedure along with the physiologic status of the patient be reported to the intensive care unit to provide continuity of care and facilitate the postoperative plan of care. The verbal report is given over the phone before the transport of the patient to the unit. The written report is given to the unit when the patient is received in the unit.

Cardiac Surgery: Nursing Procedure: Patient Transfer Report

Quality Outcome: Verbal and written reports of the intraoperative care of the cardiac surgical patient are given to the intensive care unit to provide continuity of care and facilitate the postoperative plan of care.

Performed by: Hemodynamic monitoring specialist and circulating nurse

General Statement: The verbal report is given to the unit after the patient has been weaned from cardiopulmonary bypass and is hemodynamically stable. The written documentation is completed before the transfer of the patient to the intensive care unit. The intensive care unit is notified of any delays.

Equipment: Patient transfer report sheet

Steps:	Rationale:

1. After the patient has been weaned from cardiopulmonary bypass and is hemodynamically stable, the hemodynamic monitoring specialist gives the intensive care unit a verbal intraoperative report, including but not limited to
  a. Current physiologic status of the patient
  b. Types and sites of the invasive lines
  c. Hemodynamically stabilizing drugs
  d. Implants, if applicable
  e. Ventilator settings
The hemodynamic monitoring specialist gives the ICU an approximate time of transfer.
	The verbal report facilitates the intraoperative plan of care for the patient and assists the intensive care unit with staffing.

2. The hemodynamic monitoring specialist gives the intensive care unit a report of any delays.	The hemodynamic monitoring specialist acts as a liaison with the intensive care unit. Notification of the delays assists the intensive care unit with staffing and communication with the patient's family

Steps:

3. The circulating nurse completes the transfer report before the transfer of the patient to the intensive care unit. Documentation includes but is not limited to
   a. Procedure
   b. Types of invasive lines
   c. Placement of invasive lines
   d. Blood/blood products given
   e. Blood available
   f. Urine output
   g. Cardiosupportive drug therapy
   h. Tubes/drains
   i. Temporary pacemaker leads
      1. Atrial
      2. Ventricular
   j. Weight
   k. Total body surface area
   l. Allergies
   m. Lab values
      1. Blood gases
      2. Electrolytes
      3. Hematocrit
   n. Hemodynamic pressures
      1. Cardiac output
      2. Cardiac index
      3. Arterial pressures
      4. PAD pressures
      5. CVP pressures
      6. SVR
      7. SVO_2
   o. Time of transfer
   p. Date of transfer
   q. Location of transfer
   r. Complications
   s. Special procedures and implants

Rationale:

The written report provides continuity of patient care between the two departments.

Standard of Care: Cardiac Surgery: Continuity of Care for the Immediate Postoperative Surgical Patient

I. Cardiac Surgery Reporting System
   A. Intensive care unit
      1. Verbal report
         a. Intraoperative events
         b. Current physiologic status of the patient
         c. The approximate time of arrival to the intensive care unit
      2. Written
         a. Intraoperative events
         b. Current physiologic status of the patient
         c. Arrival time and date of the patient to the intensive care unit
   B. Family
      1. Verbal report
      2. Current physiologic status of the patient
      3. The approximate time of arrival to the intensive care unit
II. Benefits of a Postoperative Reporting System
   A. Continuity of patient care
   B. Facilitates the postoperative plan of care
   C. Facilitates staffing needs
   D. Provides support for the family
III. Verbal Report
   A. The hemodynamic monitoring specialist calls the intensive care unit after the patient has been weaned from cardiopulmonary bypass and is hemodynamically stable.
      1. Information relayed
         a. Intraoperative events
         b. Current physiologic status of the patient
         c. Cardiosupportive drug therapy
         d. VADS, if applicable
         e. Ventilator settings
         f. The approximate time of transfer
   B. Communication with the family
      1. The family is supported and kept informed.
         a. The family is told the current condition of the patient.
         b. The family is told the approximate time that the patient will be in the unit.

         c. The family members are told that they will be allowed to visit as soon as the transfer has been made and the patient is stabilized.
         d. The family's questions are answered by the intensive care nurse.
IV. Written Report
    A. The circulating nurse completes the documentation sheet before the transport of the patient to the intensive care unit.
        1. Information included
            a. Procedure
            b. Types of invasive lines
            c. Placement of invasive lines
            d. Blood/blood products given
            e. Blood available
            f. Urine output
            g. Cardiosupportive drug therapy
            h. Tubes/drains
            i. Temporary pacemaker leads
                1. Atrial
                2. Ventricular
            j. Weight
            k. Total body surface area
            l. Allergies
            m. Lab values
                1. Blood gases
                2. Electrolytes
                3. Hematocrit
            n. Hemodynamic pressures
                1. Cardiac output
                2. Cardiac index
                3. Arterial pressures
                4. PAD pressures
                5. CVP pressures
                6. SVR
                7. SVO_2
            o. Time of transfer
            p. Date of transfer
            q. Location of transfer
            r. Complications
            s. Special procedures and implants
    B. The documentation sheet is taped to the front of the chart.
V. Clinical Indicators for Evaluation
    A. Feedback from the intensive care unit

      1. Pertinent information received
- B. Feedback from the family
- C. Communication between the two units
  1. Team work
- D. Continuity of care

References

American Society of Extra-Corporeal Technology. (2003). *AMSECT guidelines for perfusion practice.* Retrieved August 31, 2006, from http://www.amsect.org/general/guidelines.html.

Conner, R., & Reno, D. *AORN-association of operating room nurses standards, recommended practices, and guidelines.* (2005) Denver, CO AORN Publications.

Datascope Corporation. (2006). *Abbreviated operators guide.* Retrieved August 31, 2006, from http://www.datascope.com/ca/caedncopsguide.html.

Joint Commission of Accreditation of Healthcare Organizations, (2005). http://www.jointcommission.org.

Karp, R.B., Laks, H. & Wechsler, A.S. (1992). *Advances in cardiac surgery* St. Louis, MO. Mosby.

Occupation Safety and Health Administration. (2005) http://www.osha.gov.

Phillips, N.F. *Berry & Kohn's operating room technique.* (2003) (10th ed.). St. Louis, MO, Mosby.

Rothrock, J.C., Smith, D.A. & McEwen, D.R. *Alexander's care of the patient in surgery.* (2003) (12th ed.). St. Louis, MO, Mosby.

Spry, C. *Essentials of perioperative nursing.* (2005) MA, Jones and Bartlett Publishers.

Taylor, K.M. *Conduct of CV perfusion.* (1990) Baltimore, MD, Lippincott Williams and Wilkins.

Index

A-V loops, 181
ablation therapy, 33, 37
accountability, 99
ACLS
 certification, 25, 27, 31, 32
 coordination of, 327
 in reimplantation of cardiopulmonary bypass, 326
ACT I HPT machine, 72
ACT levels, 4
action plans
 nursing assessments and, 96
 perioperative care, 99
 revisions of, 99
activated clotting times (ACTs), 145
activity levels, assessment of, 93
adhesions, 246, 289
adipose tissue, perfusion, 157, 160, 164
admission nurses, 50–52, 53
admissions, 44, 47
adult respiratory distress syndrome, 190
adventitial pedicle, 265
agendas, staff meetings, 12
AICD. see automatic internal cardioverter defibrillator
air conduit systems, 355
alarms, 359
allergies, 60, 97, 147, 148
allergy alert bands, 53
alligator clips, 62
ambu bags, 60
American Board of Anesthesiology, 9
American Board of Surgery, 3, 9
American Board of Thoracic Surgery, 9
anesthesia
 consents, 53, 371, 372
 line supplies, 87
 nurse's role, 6
anesthesia circuits, 66
anesthesia machines, 66
anesthesia record, 377, 379
anesthesiologists
 AICD implantation, 321–322
 cardiac, 3
 during patient transfers, 250, 251–254
 in cardiopulmonary bypass, 183–189, 192, 194, 196
 in intraoperative defibrillation, 246–247
 in off-pump procedures, 214
 pacing electrode placement, 314, 315
 patient positioning and, 160
 physiologic monitoring, 129
 responsibilities, 3
 stand-by support, 57–58
 standards of care, 9
 transport of unstable patients, 109, 110–112
aneurysms, cardiothoracic, 236
annuloplasty rings, 37, 87, 230
antibiotics, preoperative, 54
anticoagulation processes, 34, 38, 185, 186
anticoagulation therapy, 182
antimicrobial solutions, 149, 154
AORN guidelines, 83, 169, 179
aorta-coronary artery bypass (CABG), 216–217
 cardiothoracic procedures, 237
 draping, 220
 indications, 218
 instrument tray, 83
 nurses' role, 6, 7
 patient history, 46
 patient positioning, 163–167, 219–220
 patient preparation, 218
 repeat procedures, 62
 room preparation, 219
 scrub nurse's role, 38
 shave prep for, 120–121, 122
 skin prep for, 152–153, 154
 standards of care, 218–225
 surgical prep, 220
aortic cross clamps, 206, 210
aortic valves, 228–235
arterial blood gases, 103, 145
arterial cannulas, 185
arterial lines, 60
arterial pressures, 33, 131
arterial spasm, 265
arterial-ventricular pacing, 61
aseptic barriers, 177
assessments. see nursing assessments; specific assessments

assistants, standard of care, 9
attendance records, 12
automatic internal cardioverter defibrillator (AICD), 320–322
autopsy forms, 341, 342
autotransfusion
   contraindications, 284
   conversion packs, 283–284
   equipment, 72, 77
   intraoperative preparation, 284–285
   machine availability, 66
   nursing procedures, 139–141
   policies, 138
   responsibility for operation, 9
   transport with, 285
autotransfusion pleural drainage units, 277, 278–286
avitiene, 62
axilla rolls, 158

backup support, scheduling of, 46
bean bags, 157, 158
beds, availability of, 43, 48
biohazardous waste, 353. see also housekeeping; waste
biological valves, 226–227
bladder catheter placement, 6
blankets, 165, 204, 214
blood. see also transfusions
   availability of, 60, 133, 219
   descending thoracic procedures, 237
   designated donor units, 133, 136
   for cardiothoracic procedures, 237
   identification of, 136
   refrigerators, 72
   refusal of, 60
   type and cross-matching, 53, 113, 136
   unused, 136
   utilization, 136–137
   utilization policies, 133
   warmers, 72
blood bank supplies
   acquisition of, 134–135
   administration of, 34
   availability of, 183
   for re-exploration procedures, 334
   refusal of blood products, 60
   responsibility for, 10
blood flow, off-pump procedures, 215

blood gas analysis machines, 72
blood glucose machines, 72
blood pressure
   cuffs, 129
   in neonates, 347
   monitors, 72
   noninvasive monitoring by, 131
   perioperative assessment of, 98
blood salvaging techniques, 137
blood urea nitrogen (BUN), 93
body bags, 344
body temperature
   after bypass, 188
   during cardiopulmonary bypass, 182
   in myocardial protection, 206
   in neonates, 346
   monitoring, 347
   monitors, 72
   noninvasive monitoring of, 131
   perfusionist's role, 5
breath sounds, 92, 98
breathing, assessment of, 92
budget management, 11–12. see also cost containment
buretrols, 347

call
   coverage, 125
   notification, 18, 20, 48
   schedules, 19
cannulation processes, 38
capillary filling, 90
cardiac catheterization, preoperative, 103
cardiac enzymes, 93
cardiac function, assessment of, 93–94
cardiac index, interpretation of, 33
cardiac managers
   documentation, 378
   monthly inservice meetings, 40–41
   monthly safety report, 350
   notification of deaths, 341, 344
   sanitation oversight, 354
   scheduling, 43–63
   standards of care, 11–13
   team mobilization by, 48, 57, 333
   team notification by, 17, 18
cardiac output monitors, 72
cardiac output, monitoring of, 131

cardiac surgeons
  consents and, 374
  draping procedures and, 170, 172–174, 175
  in cardiopulmonary bypass procedures, 183–189, 194, 196
  in IMA harvest, 267
  in internal fibrillation, 244–245
  in myocardial protection, 203, 208
  in VAD implantation, 298
  networking with, 24
  notifications of death, 344
  pacing electrode placement, 313
  preferences, 13, 191 (*see also* physician preference cards)
  pronouncements of death, 341
  responsibilities, 3
  standards of care, 9
cardiac surgery. *see also specific* policies; *specific* procedures; *specific* staff members
  nursing procedures, 18
  orientation, 29–31
  policies, 15–17, 40–41
  program dynamics, 1–13
  standard of care, 9–13
  teams, 3–13
cardiac team. *see also* anesthesiologists; cardiac managers; cardiac surgeons; circulating nurses; hemodynamic monitoring specialists; perfusionists; scrub nurses
  building of, 21–22
  contact information for, 18
  development of, 11
  efficiency of, 70
  monthly inservice meetings, 40–41
  networking, 21–24
  stand-by support, 59
  teamwork by, 22–23
cardioplegia lines, 181, 190, 205, 210, 212
cardioplegic arrest, 206
cardiopulmonary bypass cardiotomy suction, 137
cardiopulmonary bypass procedures
  anesthesiologist's role, 3–4
  descending thoracic procedures, 237
  discontinuation, 196–197
  documentation, 98, 198–200
  during valve procedures, 232
  equipment, 190–191
  expedited initiation of, 61
  femoral cannulation for, 295–296
  implementation of, 194–196
  in cardiothoracic procedures, 240
  in VAD implantation, 298
  indications, 190
  introduction to, 181–182
  nursing procedures, 183–189
  off-pump procedures, 214
  perfusionist's role, 4–5
  phases of, 190
  policies, 180
  postbypass phase, 197–198
  previous surgeries, 44
  procedures, 192
  re-exploration procedures, 336, 337
  reimplantation, 325, 326–331
  scrub nurses' role, 38
  standards of care, 190–210
  weaning the patient, 98, 270
cardiopulmonary bypass vent lines, 137
cardiosupportive drug therapy, 33, 214
cardiothoracic procedures
  draping for, 175–176, 178–179
  indications for, 236
  patient positioning for, 168
  shave prep for, 118–119, 122
  skin prep for, 150–151, 154
  standards of care, 236–242
cardiotomy suction, 181
care plans, 10, 191
case cost documentation, 87–88
case documentation, 6
case management, 65–88
  for CABG procedures, 224
  for cardiothoracic procedures, 242
  in valve procedures, 234–235
  of patient transfers, 257
  total quality management and, 124
case preparation, 240–241
catheterization laboratories, 57–58
CBP, during CABG procedures, 222
cell savers
  availability, 66
  blood salvage, 137
  connection of, 221
  operation of, 72, 138
  pleural drainage unit, 278
  reservoirs, 284
central venous pressures, 131

Index   **391**

certifications
   ACLS, 25, 27, 31, 32
   American Board of Surgery, 3
   CPR, 25, 27, 28, 31, 32
charge stickers, 86
chart reviews, 5, 33, 54, 100, 372. *see also* documentation; medical records
chemical pefusates, 211–212
chest
   draping of, 174, 176, 177, 178
   shave prep, 118, 120, 121
   x-rays, 62, 103, 289
circulating nurses. *see also* primary circulating nurses; second circulating nurses
   AICD implantation, 321–322
   autotransfusion equipment and, 139–141
   bank blood acquisition, 134
   cardiothoracic procedures, 238
   communication with patients, 54
   consents and, 374–375
   documentation by, 377
   during pacemaker insertion, 317
   during patient transfers, 250, 251–254
   IABPs placement, 310
   in autotransfusion pleural drainage units, 278–282
   in cardiopulmonary bypass, 183–189, 193, 195, 197
   in internal fibrillation, 244–245
   in intraoperative defibrillation, 246–247
   in intraoperative mortality, 344
   in myocardial protection, 203, 204, 209
   in patient transport, 52, 54, 106
   in re-exploration procedure, 337
   in re-exploration procedures, 333
   in reimplantation of cardiopulmonary bypass, 327, 330–331
   in VAD implantation, 298, 299
   instrument counts, 81, 82
   instrument inventory management, 80–81
   intra-aortic balloon placement, 305–308
   intraoperative death documentation, 343
   pacing electrode placement, 315
   patient positioning and, 157, 160, 164
   patient transfer reports, 381–382
   perioperative patient assessments, 95–96
   physiologic monitoring, 129
   preoperative lab procedures, 101–102
   proficiency skills checklist, 32–35
   protective attire, 367
   responsibilities, 5–7
   review of consents, 372, 373
   room preparation, 219, 230
   skin prep, 148–149, 150, 152–153
   stand-by support, 57–58
   transport of unstable patients, 109, 110–112, 113
circulatory system, assessment of, 93–94
clean areas, 68
cleanup times, 47
cleanup, surgical suite, 352–354
clergy, 23, 344
CLIA documentation, 143
climate control, 355
clinical indicators
   after IABPs placement, 311
   AICD implantation, 324
   autotransfusion system, 286
   continuity of care, 384–385
   documentation, 200
   education program evaluation, 31
   for CABG procedures, 224
   for cardiothoracic procedures, 242
   for documentation, 379
   for draping procedures, 179
   for electrical safety, 360
   for environmental control, 355
   for evaluation, 24, 55
   for femoral cannulation, 296
   for valve procedures, 234–235
   IMA harvesting, 272–273
   in intraoperative deaths, 345
   in myocardial protection, 213
   in reimplantation of cardiopulmonary bypass, 331
   in shave prep, 122
   inventory management, 88
   nursing assessments, 99
   of defibrillation, 249
   of patient transfers, 257–258
   of physiologic monitoring, 132
   pacemakers, 319
   patient transfers to surgery, 108
   preoperative procedures, 104
   risk management, 370
   scheduling effectiveness, 47
   surgical consent procedures, 375
   surgical skin preps, 154–155

surgical suite organization, 70–71
transfer of unstable patients, 114
VAD implantation, 301
clippers, 117
CO_2 monitors, 72
coagulation panels, preoperative, 103
cognitive function, 91, 98
cold intermittent cardioplegia, 203–207, 212
communication. *see also* patient education
   call notification, 18
   cardiac team, 67
   in cardiothoracic procedures, 240
   intraoperative plans and, 267
   nurse's role, 6
   on repeat surgical procedures, 288, 289
   patient transfers to surgery, 108
   postoperative patient transfer, 256–257
   quality indicators, 61
   responsibility for, 10
   scheduling and, 43
   scrub nurse's role, 39
   surgery reporting system, 383
   team mobilization and, 48
   total quality management and, 125
   with families, 55, 383–384
   with patients, 101
competency review, 31, 36
complete blood count (CBC), 93
computer access, 125
conduit harvesting instruments, 222
consents
   content of, 374
   for anesthesia, 53, 371, 372
   for emergent procedures, 373
   for intra-aortic balloon pumps, 302
   for observers, 375
   for photographs, 375
   for surgery, 372, 375
   for transfusions, 53, 133, 371, 372
   for transport, 109
   for universal blood/blood products, 136
   in charts, 50
   nurse responsibilities in, 374–375
   nursing procedures for, 371–373
   policies, 371
   refusal of treatment, 371, 372
   review of, 372, 373
   signed and witnessed, 53
   standards of care, 374–375

surgeon responsibilities, 374
contaminated areas, 68
continual quality improvement policies, 123
continuing education, 26, 30–31, 376, 378
continuity of care, 383–385
coping mechanisms, 99
coronary angiograms, 103, 190
coronary arteriotomy, 268
coronary artery bypass procedure, 172–174, 177–178
coronary artery obstruction, 218
coronary artherectomy, 56–58, 59–61
coronary perfusion, 60, 303
coroner, notification of, 344
cost containment, 32, 124. *see also* budget management
count sheets, 79, 80
counterpulsation, 303, 309–311
countershocks, 321
CPR (cardiopulmonary resuscitation)
   cardiopulmonary bypass initiation and, 262
   certification, 25, 27, 28, 31, 32
   documentation of, 376
   in progress, 60, 61
critical thinking, 34, 39
Cryoglue, 62
customer satisfaction, 224, 235
CVP, interpretation of, 33

data collection, responsibility for, 12–13
decannulation processes, 38, 189
defibrillation
   AICD implantation, 320
   circulating nurse's role, 33
   countershocks, 321
   external, 243
   external electrode needs, 62
   in myocardial protection, 206
   internal, 243
   intraoperative, 246–247
   myocardial damage from, 245
   nursing procedures, 244–245
   on repeat surgical procedures, 289
   standards of care, 248–249
   types of, 248
defibrillator paddles, 213
defibrillators, 66, 72, 87
dentures, removal of, 53
depression, assessment of, 92

designated cardiac call, 16
dextrose, 347
diabetes, assessment of, 91
diagnoses, procedures and, 44
diagnostic testing, 103
diaphoresis, 97
diet, assessment of, 91
disease processes, education, 53
dispersive electrode pads, 159, 363–364
displays, 72
disposition of body forms, 341
documentation
    AICDs, 320, 322, 323–324
    case costs, 87–88
    continuing education, 376
    CPR, 376
    during valve procedures, 233
    electrical safety, 356, 376
    for cardiothoracic procedures, 241–242
    housekeeping, 376
    IABPs placement, 311
    implantation, 376
    in cardiopulmonary bypass procedures, 198–200, 328, 331
    in intraoperative mortality, 341–343, 344–345
    in VAD implantation, 299
    infection control, 376
    intensive care sheets, 257
    intra-aortic balloon pumps, 302
    inventory management, 79, 376
    inventory records, 87–88
    of CABG procedures, 223
    of defibrillation, 249
    of inservice meetings, 40–41
    of nursing assessments, 96
    of pacemaker insertion, 317
    of patient positioning, 159, 162, 168
    of patient transfers, 257
    of physiologic monitoring, 132
    of shave prep, 119, 122
    of variances, 55
    operative reports, 166
    pacemakers, 319
    patient transfer reports, 253
    perioperative, 12, 376, 377–378
    policies, 376
    postoperative, 383
    preoperative checklists, 102
    procedure logs, 223–224, 233–234
    procedures, 376
    re-exploration procedures, 338
    requisitions, 85
    responsibility for, 9, 10
    safety reports, 349, 350, 360
    sanitation processes, 353
    scheduling-related, 46–47
    standards of care, 379–380
    Stat lab protocols, 142
    statistical, 376, 379
    supply logs, 84
    surgery reporting system, 383
    surgical consents, 372–373
    surgical skin preps, 149, 151, 154–155
    total quality management and, 125
    transfusion reactions, 133
    transfusions, 136
    VAD implantation, 297, 301
    valve implantation logs, 234
    work process controls, 369
dopamine, 61
drainage tubes, 222, 223, 240, 270, 278–282
drapes
    organization of, 76
draping materials
    criteria for, 177
    in myocardial protection, 204
    organization of, 172, 175
    positioning of, 177
draping procedures
    cardiothoracic procedures, 239
    during CABG procedures, 166, 216, 220–221
    during shave prep, 116
    during valve procedures, 231–232
    for cardiothoracic procedures, 175–176
    for coronary artery bypass, 172–174
    knowledge of, 37–38
    nursing procedures, 170–171
    policies, 169
    preoperative case preparation, 77
    re-exploration procedures, 335
    standards of care, 177–179
    sterile field preparation, 77
dressings, 223, 256
dysrhythmias
    induction of, 322
    interpretation of, 33
    pacemaker insertion, 316

recognition of, 37
treatment modalities, 33, 37

echocardiograms, preoperative, 103
edema, assessment of, 90, 97
education
    cardiac nursing staff, 27
    cardiac surgery programs, 25–26
    scrub nurses, 36
elective procedures
    scheduling of, 44–45, 46
    team notification of, 17
electrical conduction equipment, 72
electrical line isolation monitors, 356, 359
electrical outlets, 66
electrical safety
    documentation, 376
    policies, 356
    standards of care, 359–360
electrocardiography (EKGs)
    assessment of, 93
    courses, 28
    during patient transfer, 256
    equipment, 72
    interpretation of, 33
    noninvasive monitoring by, 131
    preoperative, 103
    transport of unstable patients, 110–112
electrocautery
    nursing procedures, 362–365
    pencils, 221, 364
    policies, 361
    safety, 34
    units, 66, 73
electrodes, placement, 129, 313–315
electrolyte analysis machines, 72
electrolytes
    assessment of, 93
    balance, 5
    stat lab capabilities, 145
electrosurgical dispersement pads, 348
emboli, prevention of, 185
emergency power systems, 356, 359–360
emergent procedures
    after trauma, 236
    consent for, 373
    patient assessments, 59–60
    scheduling, 46, 48–49
    team notification of, 17

emotional status, 54, 91, 98
emotional support, provision of, 60
endotracheal tubes, 252, 346
engineering control, 369–370
environmental control, 352–354, 355
environmental precautions, 125
epicardial pacemaker leads, 72
epinephrine, 61
equipment
    cardiac surgical suites, 66
    for cardiopulmonary bypass, 190–191
    inspection of, 359
    inventory records, 87–88
    maintenance logs, 12
    organization of, 68
    positioning of, 71
    preparation, 32
    preventive maintenance, 146, 358
    repeat procedures, 62
    scheduling of, 47
    scrub nurses' role, 37
    standards of care, 72–73
    surgical suite organization, 69, 70
evidence-based medicine, 22
extracorporal circuits, 325, 327
extracorporal table circuits, 38
extracorporeal circulation, 4, 182, 201
extremities, assessment of, 90
eye shields, 366, 367, 369
eyeware, protective, 367

face masks, 366, 369
facilities management, 125
families/next of kin
    communication with, 55, 113, 215, 240, 257, 289
    education of, 53
    grieving process, 345
    networking with, 23
    notification of death, 341, 344
    of neonates, 348
    postmortem visitations, 342
    preoperative education, 50
    reports to, 383–384
    support for, 340
fear, presence of, 60
felt sheets, 62
femoral arteries
    access to, 163

femoral arteries (*Continued*)
    cannulation of, 182, 292–294
    cardiopulmonary bypass via, 61
    exposure of, 294
    shave prep, 118
femoral bypass, 236, 237, 240
femoral cannulation trays, 61, 62, 83
femoral perfusion cannulas, 62
femoral region, draping of, 177, 178
femoral veins
    cannulation of, 182, 293–296
    cardiopulmonary bypass via, 61
fiberoptic headlights, 73
fibrillation, after bypass, 188
fingers, clubbing of, 90
fluid flow sheets, 377, 379
fluid lines, preparation, 32
fluid utilization sheets, 12
fluid volume replacement, 5, 347
fluids, administration of, 34
Foley catheters, 60, 113, 256
Frazier suction tips, 212

Gelfoam, 62
glasses, removal of, 53
gloves
    disposable, 369
    during shave prep, 117, 118, 119
    handling blood products, 136
    nursing procedure, 367
    policies, 366
    shave prep, 121
glucose control, 5, 145, 347
Gott shunts, 87, 237, 240
gowns, 53, 366, 367, 369
grafts
    anastomoses, 216
    handling of, 37
grieving process, 345
grounding pads, 361

hair. *see also* shave prep
    indications for removal of, 122
    insulation by, 363
hair clippers, 118
hand washing, 370
harvesting instruments, 71
hearing aids, removal of, 53
heart rates, in neonates, 347

heart sounds, assessment of, 93, 98
heart team, notification of, 12
heart-lung machines, 72, 137
    availability, 66
    cardiopulmonary bypass, 180, 181–182, 190
    cleaning of, 189
    maintenance of, 200
    perfusionist's role, 4
    preparation of, 219
    scrub nurses' role, 36
heat loss, in neonates, 348
heating blankets, 214
hematocrits, 145
hemoconcentration systems, 72, 137, 210
hemodynamic monitoring
    application of equipment, 55
    during transport, 105
    transport of unstable patients, 109
hemodynamic monitoring specialists
    cardiothoracic procedures, 239
    during patient transfers, 250, 251–254
    in cardiopulmonary bypass, 183–189, 197
    in intraoperative defibrillation, 246–247
    intra-aortic balloon placement, 306, 308
    pacing electrode placement, 313
    perioperative patient assessments, 95–96
    physiologic monitoring, 129
    protective attire, 367
    room preparation, 219, 230
    stand-by support, 57–58
    standards of care, 9
    transport of unstable patients, 110–112, 113
hemodynamics, interpretation, 33, 37
hemorrhages, postoperative, 332–339
heparin, 182, 185, 219
heparin dose response (HDR), 145
heparin protamine titration (HPT), 145
heparinization, reversal of, 330
hepatitis B vaccination, 369
homeostasis, 62, 290
housekeeping
    documentation, 376, 378
    documentation logs, 12
    policies, 351
    protocols, 125
    risk management and, 370
    schedules, 355
housekeeping manager, 354
hyperlipidemia, assessment of, 93

hypertension, assessment of, 93
hypothermia, 206

identification bands, 53
implant logs, 378
implantation documentation, 376
implanted devices, 60, 72, 87, 229
infection control
   circulating nurse's role, 34
   documentation, 376, 378
   draping procedures and, 170–171, 172–174
   housekeeping and, 351
   monthly inservice meetings, 31
   protective attire, 366
   shave prep and, 122
   surgical skin prep and, 150
   surgical suite, 352–354
   surgical suite organization and, 71
   total quality management and, 125
   traffic patterns and, 68
   work process controls, 369
infection rates, 224, 234
infections, susceptibility to, 54
informed consent, 136. *see also* consents
infusion pumps, 66
inservice meetings, 30–31, 40, 350, 369
instrument inventory management, 82–83, 83
instrument room personnel, 80–81
instrument trays
   organization of, 79, 82
   positioning of, 75, 76
instruments
   counts, 6, 10, 11, 82, 219, 223, 233, 240
   damaged, 80
   inspection of, 80
   inventory management, 79, 80–81
   organization of, 11
   sterilization, 82
insulin, use of, 182
insurance, carrier names, 50
integumentary status, 90
intensive care documentation sheets, 376, 378, 379
intensive care emergency chest set, 83
intensive care units
   after CABG procedures, 223
   autotransfusion system in, 285–286
   communication with, 48, 240, 250, 257
   notification of deaths, 344
   patient transport to, 339
intercostal arteries, 265
interdepartmental networking, 23, 108, 113
internal defibrillators, 87
internal mammary arteries (IMAs)
   contraindications to grafting, 271
   harvesting, 37, 222, 264–266, 271–273
   harvesting equipment, 271–272
   location, 271
   nursing procedures, 267–270
   utilization of, 271
intra-aortic balloon pumps (IABPs), 72
   console maintenance, 311
   contraindications, 303–304
   counterpulsation using, 309–311
   monitoring, 310
   nursing procedures, 304
   policies, 302
   responsibility for, 9
   use of, 61
   utilization, 303–304
intra-aortic balloons, 72, 305–308
intraluminal synthetic vascular grafts, 87
intraoperative blood salvaging techniques, 137
intraoperative defibrillation, 246–247
intraoperative monitoring, 3, 37
intraoperative mortalities, 340–345
invasive lines
   notation of, 60
   placement, 9, 130, 219, 256
   preparation, 33
invasive monitoring, 127, 131, 220, 239
inventory management
   documentation, 376, 378
   instruments, 79, 80–81, 82–83
   requisitions, 85–86
   responsibility for, 12
   standards of care, 87–88
   supplies, 84
irrigation, 210, 348
isolated power systems, 357
isolettes, 346
IV fluids, 9
IV lines, 5

JCAHO, documentation for, 378
job performance evaluations, 11, 31

K-thermia blankets, 187, 206
K-thermia machines, 66, 212

laboratory procedures
   assessment of, 93
   for off-pump procedures, 214
   invasive monitoring of, 132
   physiologic monitoring, 128
   preoperative, 100–102, 103
   results in charts, 50, 53
lamps, 66–67, 73. *see also* lighting
language barriers, 91
laundry, 353, 368, 370
left ventricular pressures, 131
leg holders, 165
legs, shave prep, 118, 120
lengths of stay, 50
levels of activity, 91
levels of comprehension, 91
levels of consciousness, 54, 91
levophed, 61
licensed personnel, 19
   cardiac nursing staff, 27
   educational requirements, 19, 30
   entry level, 25
   teamwork approach, 22
licensure, 31, 146
lidocaine, 61
lifts, availability, 66
lighting, 73. *see also* lamps
   cardiac surgical suites, 66–67
   during shave prep, 116, 119, 120
   emergency, 67
lot numbers, recall notifications and, 86
lower extremities, draping of, 177–178
LVAD/RVAD, 61

Marfan's syndrome, 236
mayo stands
   movement of, 222
   organization of, 219
   placement of, 71, 76, 78, 165, 220, 221
   positioning, 161
mechanical assistive devices, 60, 72
mechanical valves, 226
mechanical ventilation, 109
medial degeneration, 236
median sternotomy, 77
mediastinal autotransfusion system, 283

mediastinal drainage system, 283, 334
mediastinum, re-exploration, 332–339
medical assist devices, 72
medical diagnoses, assessment of, 97
medical examiner's case criteria, 341
medical examiners, 341, 345
medical history. *see* patient history
medical records, 50, 53. *see also* chart reviews
medical-legal issues, 124
mentation, assessment of, 91, 93
mitral valves, 228–235
mixed venous saturation, 33, 131
mobility, assessment of, 97
monitoring equipment, 55, 72
monitoring, patient positioning and, 156
monitors, 72
monthly meetings, 40–41
morgue packs, 341, 342
morgue, transport to, 342, 344
mortalities, 23, 340–345, 341
mortality risk documentation sheets, 377, 379
mortuary release forms, 341
motor impairments, 54, 90
myocardial protection
   chemical pefusates, 211–212
   cold intermittent cardioplegia, 203–207
   during CABG procedures, 222
   goals, 211
   nursing procedures, 203–207, 208–210
   phases of, 211
   standards of care, 211–213
   types of, 211
   valve procedures, 232
   warm continuous cardioplegia, 208–210
myocardial protection techniques
   introduction to, 181–182
   knowledge of, 34, 38
   policies, 202
   use of, 187
myocardial revascularization, 214
myocardium
   damage due to defibrillation, 247
   ischemic, 218
   revascularization of, 218

narcotics, preoperative, 51, 54
neck vein distention, 90
needles
   counting of, 6, 10, 11, 223

handling of, 369
neonates, 346–348
networking
  cardiac team, 21–24
  circulating nurse's role in, 32
  encouragement of, 26
  for cardiothoracic procedures, 242
  in CABG procedures, 225
  in valve procedures, 235
  total quality management and, 124
noninvasive monitoring
  application of equipment, 55, 60
  cardiothoracic procedures, 239
  circulating nurse's role, 33
  components of, 127
  during pacemaker insertion, 316–317
  during patient transport, 107
  during valve procedures, 231
  equipment placement, 219
  nurse's role, 5, 6
  patient transfers to surgery, 108
  re-exploration procedures, 335
  transport of unstable patients, 110–112
  types of, 131
nonlicensed personnel, 19, 22, 25, 28
normal thermia, 214
notifications of death, 344
NPO status, verification of, 54
nurses. *see also* circulating nurses; scrub nurses
  call notification, 18
  educational requirements, 27, 28
  patient transfers, 106–107
  perioperative function of, 97
  shave prep by, 116
  standards of care, 9–10
nursing assessments
  care plans and, 262
  circulating nurse's role, 33
  completion of, 54
  during patient transfers, 252
  IABPs placement, 310
  in charts, 53
  in emergent procedures, 60
  in transfers to surgery, 106–107
  intra-aortic balloon pumps and, 304
  neonates, 346–347
  patient positioning and, 160, 162, 164, 167
  perioperative, 89–99
  preoperative, 54

skin, 364–365
  total quality management and, 125
nursing assistants, 106–107, 116
nursing care plans, 54, 125
nursing procedures
  AICD implantation, 321–322
  assessment of lab procedures, 101–102
  autotransfusion, 139–141
  autotransfusion pleural drainage units, 278–282
  bank blood acquisition, 134–135
  draping, 170–171, 175–176
  electrical hazard prevention, 357–358
  electrocautery safety, 362–365
  environmental control, 352–354
  femoral artery cannulation, 293–294
  IMA harvesting, 267–270
  institution of cardiopulmonary bypass, 183–189
  instrument inventory management, 80–81
  internal defibrillation, 244–245
  intra-aortic balloon placement, 305–308
  intraoperative defibrillation, 246–247
  maintenance of the Stat lab, 143–144
  monthly inservice meetings, 41
  myocardial protection, 203–207, 208–210
  pacemaker insertion, 316–317
  pacing electrode placement, 313–315
  patient positioning and, 157–159, 160–162, 164–166
  patient transfer reports, 381–382
  patient transfer to surgery, 106–107
  perioperative assessments, 95–96
  perioperative documentation, 377–378
  physiologic monitoring, 129–130
  postoperative patient transfers, 251–254
  protective attire, 367–368
  re-exploration procedures, 333–336
  reimplantation of cardiopulmonary bypass, 326–328
  repeat surgical procedures, 288–289
  safety reports, 350
  same-day admissions, 50–52
  scheduling emergent procedures, 48–49
  shave prep, 118–119, 120–121
  skin prep, 152–153
  slush machines, 275–276
  sterile field preparation, 75–76
  surgical consents, 371–373

nursing procedures (*Continued*)
  surgical suite organization, 69
  transport of unstable patients, 110–112
  VAD implantation, 298–299
nursing process, 30, 34, 39
nutritional status, 91, 93, 97

observers, consent for, 375
office coordinators, 50–52
on-call teams, 16
open sores, assessment of, 91
operating hours, scheduled, 47
operating rooms. *see* surgical suites
operative record, responsibility for, 12
orderlies, 106–107, 116
orientation manuals, 29, 125
orientation process
  preceptors and, 25–26
  standards of care, 29–31
  steps in, 29
  total quality management and, 124
oscillating saws, 62
outcomes, documentation of, 55
oxygen saturation, 103, 346
oxygen therapy
  during transport, 105
  retinopathy of prematurity and, 346
  transport of unstable patients, 109
oxyhemoglobin, monitoring of, 131

pacemakers
  electrode placement, 318
  indications, 318
  permanent, 87, 316–317
  standards of care, 318–319
  system selection, 318
pacing catheters, 60
pacing therapy, 33, 37
pacing wires, 213, 256
pacing, policies, 312
pain
  assessment of, 54, 92
  control of, 60
  perioperative assessment of, 98
  presence of, 60
papaverine, 265, 268
pathology, specimens to, 232
patient education
  circulating nurse's role, 33

evaluation of, 55
for CABG procedures, 224
in valve procedures, 235
preoperative, 50, 53, 54
questions answered, 54
patient history
  assessment of, 92
  in charts, 50, 53
  preoperative, 102, 103, 104
  previous surgeries, 44–45
  scheduling and, 46
patient identification
  by admissions nurse, 53
  circulating nurse's role, 33
  confirmation of, 51
  preoperative lab procedures, 101
  responsibility for, 10
  transport of unstable patients, 113
patient positioning
  CABG procedures, 163, 164–166, 219–220
  circulating nurse's role, 34
  criteria for, 167
  descending thoracic procedures, 237, 238
  during shave prep, 119
  electrode positioning and, 363
  for cardiothoracic procedures, 237
  indications, 300
  nurse's role, 6
  nursing procedures, 157–159
  policies, 156
  re-exploration procedures, 335, 338
  standards of care, 167–168
  valve procedures, 231
patient transport
  after CABG procedures, 223
  after cardiothoracic procedures, 241
  after IABPs placement, 311
  after valve procedures, 233
  counting of, 11
  nurse's role, 5
  nursing procedures, 106–107
  physiologic monitoring during, 130
  postoperative, 250–258
  preoperative, 52, 54
  reports, 253, 380, 381–382
  responsibility for, 10
  to surgery, 105
  to the intensive care unit, 339

unstable patients, 109–114, 338
  with autotransfusion systems, 285
patients
  care activities, 105–125
  information on, 44–45
  intake procedures, 53
  physical assessments, 90–94
  quality of care, 125
  safety of, 34, 38
  special needs, 44
  stabilization of, 255
pay for performance, 31
pediatric patients, 62. *see also* neonates
peer review, 31
percutaneous transluminal coronary angioplasty (PTCA), 46, 56–58, 59–61, 259–261
performance reviews, 124
perfusion cannulas, 190
perfusion protocols, 180, 191
perfusion records, 377, 379
perfusionists
  cardiothoracic procedures, 239
  in cardiopulmonary bypass procedures, 183–189, 192, 194–195, 196–197
  in myocardial protection, 203, 205, 209
  in off-pump procedures, 214
  in reimplantation of cardiopulmonary bypass, 325, 328, 329
  in VAD implantation, 297, 298, 299
  intra-aortic balloon placement, 306, 308
  perioperative patient assessments, 95–96
  re-exploration procedures, 334
  responsibilities, 4–5, 143–144
  room preparation, 219, 230–231
  stand-by support, 57–58
  standards of care, 9
perineal area, shave prep, 118, 120
perioperative care, 99
perioperative case documentation, 12, 376
perioperative plan of care, 10, 191
perioperative surgical checklists, 379
peripheral pulses, 91
personal effects, handling of, 54
personal protective equipment, 353
photographs, consent for, 375
physical appearance, assessment of, 93
physical assessments
  cardiac surgical patients, 90–94
  in charts, 50

physical exams, preoperative, 103, 104
physician assistants, 9
physician orders, 115, 118, 120
physician preference cards, 77, 80
physicians, special needs, 44
physiologic monitoring
  during CABG procedures, 220
  lab values, 128
  nursing procedures, 129–130
  policies, 127–128
  re-exploration procedures, 336
  standards of care, 131–132
physiological assessments, 97–98
physiological status, 89, 113, 255
planning, circulating nurse's role, 34
plasma, availability, 62
platelets, availability, 62
pledgeted sutures, 62
pleural drainage, 252, 253
pleural drainage units, 277, 278–282
policies
  AICD implantation, 320
  autotransfusion, 138
  autotransfusion pleural drainage units, 277
  blood utilization, 133
  cardiopulmonary bypass, 180
  continual quality improvement, 123
  documentation, 376, 378
  draping procedures, 169
  electrical safety, 356
  electrocautery utilization, 361
  femoral artery cannulation, 292
  housekeeping, 351
  IMA harvesting, 264
  internal defibrillation, 243
  intra-aortic balloon pumps, 302
  intraoperative mortalities, 340
  myocardial protection techniques, 202
  pacing, 312
  patient positioning, 156, 160, 163
  patient transfer reports, 380
  patient transfer to surgery, 105
  perioperative documentation, 376
  physiologic monitoring, 127–128
  postoperative patient transfer, 250
  protective attire, 366
  re-exploration procedures, 332
  reimplantation of cardiopulmonary bypass, 325

Index 401

policies (*Continued*)
   repeat surgical procedures, 287
   safety reports, 349
   slush machines, 274
   Stat lab protocols, 142
   sterile field preparation, 74–78
   supply inventories, 84
   surgical consents, 371
   surgical shave prep, 115
   surgical skin prep, 147
   total quality management and, 124
   transfer of unstable patients, 109
   ventricular assist devices, 297
postmortem care, 342, 344, 345
postoperative expectations, 53
postoperative phase
   circulating nurses role, 34
   hemorrhages, 332–339
   scrub nurse's role, 39
   sterile field procedures, 78
   surgical suite organization in, 71
preceptor programs, 29
preceptors, 25–26, 30
preference cards, 13, 77, 80
preoperative medications, 54
preoperative orders, 50, 53
preoperative phase
   circulating nurse's role in, 32–33
   lab procedures, 100–102
   lab work, 50
   patient preparation, 218, 229
   plans, 60
   preparation, 89–104
   scrub nurses' role, 36
preparation time, monitoring of, 47
pressure monitors, 72
primary circulating nurses, 5–6, 9–10, 22. *see also* circulating nurses; second circulating nurses
primary scrub nurses, 11. *see also* scrub nurses
prioritization, 96, 110–112, 113, 255
privacy, during shave prep, 116, 120
problem solving, 22
procedure logs, 12, 223–224, 233–234, 241–242, 377
procedures, 13. *see also specific* procedures
   documentation, 376, 378
   total quality management and, 124
productivity, teamwork and, 22

proficiency skills checklist, 32–35
proficiency testing, 36–39, 145–146
pronouncements of death, 341, 344
prostheses, 53, 60
prosthetics, assessment of, 97
protamine, 182, 188, 330
protective attire, 366, 367–368, 369
psychosocial status, 89, 98–99
PT/PTT, assessment of, 93
PTCA. *see* percutaneous transluminal coronary angioplasty
pulmonary artery pressures, 33
pulmonary capillary wedge pressures, 33
pulmonary function testing, 103
pulse generators, 62, 72, 318
pulse oximetry, 72, 103, 129
pulses, assessment of, 93, 98
purchasing departments, 86
purse-string stitches, 185
purse-string sutures, 38

quality control
   data collection, 55
   stat lab programs, 145
   stat lab protocols, 142
quality improvement
   circulating nurse's role in, 32
   scrub nurse's role, 36
   sterile field preparation, 78
quality indicators
   atherectomy surgical support, 263
   blood salvage, 137
   for instrument inventory management, 83
   of patient positioning, 168
   percutaneous transluminal coronary angioplasty, 263
   re-exploration procedures, 339
   repeat procedures, 63
   standby-support, 61
   stenting procedures, 263
   surgical suite organization, 71
quality management
   responsibility for, 12
   standards of care and, 124–125

radial artery grafts, 265
radial artery harvesting, 163, 216, 221
radiography, 62, 103, 289
Ray-Tec sponges, 265

razors, 117
re-exploration, mediastinal, 332–339
re-operations. *see* repeat surgical procedures
recall notifications, 86
record keeping, 125. *see also* documentation
rectal probes, 347
refusal of consents, 371
refusal of treatment, 372, 373
regulatory compliance, 124
repeat surgical procedures, 62–63, 289
    case preparation, 290
    nursing procedures, 288–289
    policies, 287
    standards of care, 290–291
requisitions, for supplies, 85–86
respiratory status, assessment of, 54, 92–93, 97
restocking supplies, 34
retinopathy of prematurity, 346
revascularization procedures
    cardiopulmonary bypass and, 182
    emergent, 59–61, 261–262
    myocardial, 218
Ringer's solution, lactated, 347
risk management, 349–385
    circulating nurse's role, 34
    engineering control, 369–370
    scrub nurse's role, 39
    total quality management and, 125
    work practice controls, 369
room assessment, 5

safety
    documentation, 378
    during patient transport, 107
    electrical, 356
    electrical hazard prevention, 357–358
    for off-pump procedures, 214
    in defibrillation, 248
    monthly inservice meetings, 31
    patient positioning, 156, 167
    reports, 349
    surgical skin preps, 154
    surgical suite organization, 70
    total quality management and, 125
    transfer of unstable patients, 109
    transport of unstable patients, 110–112
safety committees, 350
safety reports, 13, 350, 360
safety straps, 129, 158

same-day admissions, 50–55
saphenous veins
    during CABG procedures, 216
    exposure of, 163, 173, 220
    grafts, 265
    harvesting, 174, 221
scars
    assessment of, 91
    insulation by, 363
scheduling, 43–63
    atherectomy surgical support, 261–263
    cardiac surgical procedures, 46–47
    clinical indicators of effectiveness, 47
    emergent procedures, 48–49
    housekeeping, 355
    information needed, 46–47
    monthly cleanings, 354
    percutaneous transluminal coronary angioplasty, 261–263
    repeat procedures, 62
    stand-by support, 59
    stenting procedures, 261–263
    surgical support, 56–58
    total quality management and, 125
scrub nurses/techs
    AICD implantation, 321–322
    autotransfusion equipment and, 139–141
    cannulation and, 185, 186, 293–294
    cardiothoracic procedures, 239
    circulating nurse's role, 32
    draping procedures and, 170–175
    during CABG procedures, 216
    during pacemaker insertion, 317
    IABPs placement, 310
    in cardiopulmonary bypass procedures, 183–189, 193–197
    in internal fibrillation, 244–245
    in myocardial protection, 203–209
    in reimplantation of cardiopulmonary bypass, 328, 329–330
    in VAD implantation, 298
    instrument counts, 81, 82
    instrument inventory management, 80–81
    intra-aortic balloon placement, 305–308
    pacing electrode placement, 313, 314
    patient positioning and, 166
    perioperative patient assessments, 95–96
    preoperative case preparation, 77
    proficiency skills, 36–39

scrub nurses/techs (*Continued*)
   protective attire, 367
   re-exploration procedures, 334, 335, 336
   responsibilities, 6–8
   room preparation, 219, 230–231
   stand-by support, 57–58
   sterility field preparation, 75–76
   teamwork approach, 22–23
   valve procedures, 232
second circulating nurses. *see also* circulating nurses; primary circulating nurses
   in reimplantation of cardiopulmonary bypass, 328
   responsibilities, 6–7
   standards of care, 10–11
   teamwork approach, 22
sensory impairments, 54, 90, 98
sharps, handling of, 369
shave prep
   circulating nurse's role, 33
   for CABG, 120–121
   for cardiothoracic procedures, 118–119
   for valve procedures, 116–117
   in emergent procedures, 60
   policies, 115
   preoperative, 54
   standards of care, 122
   timing of, 51
   unstable patients, 113
shoe covers, 366, 369
sitting stools, 66
skills checklists, 124
skin
   assessment of, 90, 93, 97, 118, 120, 149, 364–365
   preoperative, 54
skin prep, 10, 34, 147–155
slush machines, 73, 182
   availability, 66
   in myocardial protection, 212
   placement of, 221
   policies, 274
   positioning, 240
   preparation, 219
   valve procedures, 232
special orders' logs, 12
specimen handling, 370
sponges, counting of, 6, 10, 11, 223
staff
   development, 124

grieving process, 345
staff education
   documentation, 379
   electrical safety, 359
   for CABG procedures, 224
   for environmental control, 355
   in cardiopulmonary bypass, 191
   in defibrillation, 248
   in electrical safety, 362
   in equipment maintenance, 73
   in equipment use, 73
   in valve procedures, 235
staff meetings, 11, 12
staff scheduling, 11, 19
staffing issues
   call notification, 18
   call time, 19
   clinical indicators, 20
   designated cardiac call, 16
   regular time hours, 19
   standards of care, 19–20
   surgical suite staff, 15
   team notification, 17
stand-by coverage, 57–58
stand-by support, 59–61
standardization, 23, 87
standards of care
   AICD implantation, 323–324
   aorta-coronary artery bypass (CABG), 218–225
   atherectomy surgical support, 261–263
   autotransfusion pleural drainage units, 283–286
   blood utilization, 136–137
   cardiac surgery, 9–13
   cardiac surgery orientation, 29–31
   cardiac surgical equipment, 72–73
   cardiac surgical team, 9–13
   cardiac team networking, 21–24
   cardiopulmonary bypass, 190–210
   cardiothoracic procedures, 236–242
   competency reviews, 31
   continuity of care, 383–385
   counterpulsation, 309–311
   defibrillation, 248–249
   draping, 177–179
   electrical safety, 359–360
   environmental control, 355
   femoral cannulation, 295–296

IMA harvesting, 271–273
implementation of, 99
in intraoperative mortality, 344–345
in myocardial protection, 211–213
in reimplantation of cardiopulmonary bypass, 329–331
instrument inventory management, 82–83
inventory management, 87–88
knowledge of, 34
pacemakers, 318–319
patient positioning, 167–168
patient transfers to surgery, 108
percutaneous transluminal coronary angioplasty, 261–263
perioperative documentation, 379–380
perioperative nursing assessments, 97–99
physiologic monitoring, 131–132
postoperative patient transfers, 255–258
preoperative procedures, 103–104
proficiency skills, 36–39
re-exploration procedures, 337–339
repeat procedures, 62–63
repeat surgical procedures, 290–291
responsibility for, 13
same-day admissions, 53–55
scrub nurse's role, 39
staffing for cardiac procedures, 19–20
Stat labs, 145–146
stenting procedures, 261–263
sterile field preparation, 77–78
surgical consents, 374–375
surgical shave preps, 122
surgical skin preps, 154–155
surgical suite organization, 70–71
total quality management and, 124–125
transport of unstable patients, 113–115
VAD implantation, 300–301
valve procedures, 228–235
standby-support, 61
standing stools, 73
stat labs
    capabilities, 145
    cardiopulmonary bypass and, 191
    equipment, 4, 72
    maintenance, 143–144
    protocols, 142
    re-exploration procedures, 336
    standards of care, 145–146
statistical documentation, 376
stenting procedures, 56–61, 190, 259–263
sterile field preparation, 37, 74–78, 169
sterilization, instruments, 82
sternal rewiring trays, 83
sternal saws, 77, 221
sternotomy, 205, 209, 221
storage, 72, 136
strategic planning, 23
stress levels, 98–99
suite cleanup, 34
supine positioning, 161, 165
supplies
    descending thoracic procedures, 237
    in cardiothoracic procedures, 236–237
    inventory, 84
    inventory records, 87–88
    location of, 67
    organization of, 68
    requisitions, 85–86
    standardization of, 87
    Stat labs, 146
    surgical suite organization, 69
supply logs, 84, 85
support mechanisms, 23
supportive drug therapy, 60, 61, 262, 263
surgeons. *see* cardiac surgeons
surgery reporting system, 383
surgery, consent for, 372, 374–375
surgical case logs, 379
surgical plans, 53
surgical prep, 231, 293, 300–301
surgical records, 377, 378, 379
surgical suites
    assessment, 5
    designated, 65–88
    environmental control, 346, 352–354, 355
    housekeeping, 351
    organization of, 68–71
    preparation, 10, 32, 37, 219, 230–231, 238
    stand-by availability, 59
    surgical team, 15
surgical supplies, 12
surgical tables, transfer to, 114
surgical team, introduction, 29
surgical time, actual, 47
surgicele, 62
sutures, knowledge of, 37
SVO_2 monitors, 72
SVR, interpretation of, 33

Index 405

Swan-Ganz catheters, 60, 165
Swan-Ganz lines, 161

tape, patient positioning and, 159
team building, 21–22
team education
    repeat procedures, 62–63
    repeat surgical procedures, 290–291
teamwork, 22–23, 26
technical competency check list, 29
temperature control, 60, 107, 212
thermia units, 73
thoracic trays, 83
thrombin, 62
time management, 83
tissue perfusion, 157
total quality management, 124–125
tourniquets, 185
towels. *see* draping materials
traffic patterns, 68, 71
training, exposure control and, 369
transducers, 9
transfusions. *see also* blood; blood bank supplies
    consent forms, 53
    consents, 133, 371, 372
    documentation, 136
    reactions, 133, 137
transport humidifiers, 346
transport monitors, 72
trends analysis, 379
tricuspid valves, 228–235
turnover times, 47

ulnar nerves, 165
ulnar pads, 220
ultrafiltration, 191
unit nurses, 113
unstable patients
    surgical skin prep for, 148, 150, 152
    transfer to surgery, 109–114, 338
urine output, 131, 253

vacuum-assisted positioning devices, 215
valve graft conduits, 87
valve implantation logs, 234
valve procedures
    draping for, 170, 178
    indications, 228

instrument tray, 83
inventories, 87
patient history, 46
patient positioning, 160–162, 167–168
previous surgeries, 44–45
room preparation, 230–231
shave prep for, 116–, 122
skin prep for, 148–149, 154
standards of care, 228–235
types, 226
valve sizes, 230
valve/implant logs, 12
valves
    biological, 226–227
    implants, 229
    incompetent, 226
    inventories, 87
    mechanical, 226
    repair *versus* replacement, 228–229
    stenotic, 226
valvular heart disease, 228
variances, documentation of, 13, 376, 378
vascular conduits, 44, 221, 222
vein harvesting tray, 83, 221
vena cava compression, 186
venous blood gases, 145
vent circuits, 181
ventilators, presence of, 60
ventricular assist devices
    indications, 300
    LVAD/RVAD, 61, 301
    nursing procedures, 298–299
    policies, 297
    standards of care, 300–301
    types of, 300
ventricular irritability, 130
verbal reports, 383
vericose veins, 91
vital signs, preoperative, 54
vitamin K, 347

warm continuous cardioplegia, 208–210, 212
warranties, for instruments, 83
waste
    disposal, 353, 368
    removal protocols, 355
weight, assessment of, 91
work practice controls, 369